MRSA

MRSA
SECOND EDITION

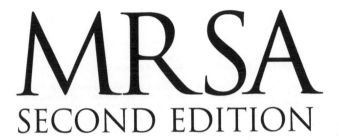

EDITED BY
JOHN A. WEIGELT, M.D.
MEDICAL COLLEGE OF WISCONSIN
DIVISION OF TRAUMA AND CRITICAL CARE
DEPARTMENT OF SURGERY
MILWAUKEE, WISCONSIN, USA

informa
healthcare

New York London

Informa Healthcare USA, Inc.
52 Vanderbilt Avenue
New York, NY 10017

© 2010 by Informa Healthcare USA, Inc.
Informa Healthcare is an Informa business

No claim to original U.S. Government works

10 9 8 7 6 5 4 3 2 1

International Standard Book Number-10: 1-4398-1879-7 (Softcover)
International Standard Book Number-13: 978-1-4398-1879-4 (Softcover)

Library of Congress Cataloging-in-Publication Data

MRSA / edited by John A. Weigelt. — 2nd ed.
    p. ; cm.
  Includes bibliographical references and index.
  ISBN-13: 978-1-4398-1879-4 (softcover : alk. paper)
  ISBN-10: 1-4398-1879-7 (softcover : alk. paper) 1. Staphylococcus aureus infections–Chemotherapy. 2. Methicillin resistance. I. Weigelt, John A.
  [DNLM: 1. Staphylococcal Infections–prevention & control. 2. Community-Acquired Infections–prevention & control. 3. Cross Infection–prevention & control. 4. Methicillin Resistance. 5. Methicillin-Resistant Staphylococcus aureus–drug effects. WC 250 M9385 2009]

    QR201.S68M77 2009
    616.9'297—dc22

                                                    2009037785

For Corporate Sales and Reprint Permissions call 212-520-2700 or write to: Sales Department, 52 Vanderbilt Avenue, 7th floor, New York, NY 10017.

**Visit the Informa Web site at
www.informa.com**

**and the Informa Healthcare Web site at
www.informahealthcare.com**

Preface

MRSA continues to be in the medical and public headlines. New information and clarification of old information are occurring in the medical literature on a daily basis. This is exemplified by the need to rapidly update the first edition. Despite the first edition being published in 2008, we felt that enough new information regarding MRSA had become available and that a second edition was essential and required. All authors agreed with a very rapid turnaround time for each of their chapters and all achieved their goals. This second edition has been compiled within nine months, providing the reader with the latest up-to-date ground-breaking information in the field.

Each day it seems I am confronted with another patient with MRSA disease. Additionally, infection control practices are being rewritten as MRSA continues to increase within medical communities. We have added new chapters that address the new concerns raised by MRSA and its myriad of presentations and challenges. These new chapters include a review of device infections, a discussion of MRSA resistance, and another with current information on preventive measures. All other chapters have been updated and collated keeping the information consistent and current.

Once again, I sincerely thank all the authors who were kind enough to contribute to this text. I believe we have a concise book aimed at helping clinicians everywhere understand MRSA and its ramifications. I still believe that MRSA is not completely understood by any of us. Attempting to get current information into the hands of clinicians who face these problems everyday seems to be the best way to serve our patients and our health care communities.

John A. Weigelt

Contents

Contributors

David G. Armstrong   Department of Surgery, University of Arizona College of Medicine, Tucson, Arizona, U.S.A.

Nicholas J. Bevilacqua   Amputation Prevention Center, Valley Presbyterian Hospital, Los Angeles, California, U.S.A.

Karen J. Brasel   Department of Surgery, Medical College of Wisconsin, Milwaukee, Wisconsin, U.S.A.

Jack E. Brown   State University of New York at Buffalo, Buffalo, New York, U.S.A.

Melissa Brunsvold   Department of Surgery, University of Michigan Health System, Ann Arbor, Michigan, U.S.A.

Amy E. Bryant   Infectious Diseases Section, Veterans Affairs Medical Center, Boise, Idaho, and Department of Medicine, University of Washington School of Medicine, Seattle, Washington, U.S.A.

Kent Crossley   Department of Medicine, Veterans Affairs Medical Center, and the University of Minnesota Medical School, Minneapolis, Minnesota, U.S.A.

Jeremy Dengler   Albany College of Pharmacy and Health Sciences, Albany, New York, U.S.A.

Charles E. Edmiston, Jr.   Department of Surgery and Pathology, Medical College of Wisconsin, Milwaukee, Wisconsin, U.S.A.

Barry C. Fox   Department of Medicine, University of Wisconsin School of Medicine, University of Wisconsin Hospital and Clinics, and William S. Middleton Veterans Affairs Medical Center, Madison, Wisconsin, U.S.A.

Mary Beth Graham Division of Infectious Diseases, Department of Medicine, Medical College of Wisconsin, Milwaukee, Wisconsin, U.S.A.

Kamal M. F. Itani Boston Veterans Affairs Health Care System, Boston University, Boston, Massachusetts, U.S.A.

Anna P. Lam Division of Pulmonary and Critical Care Medicine, Northwestern University Feinberg School of Medicine, Chicago, Illinois, U.S.A.

Nathan A. Ledeboer Department of Surgery and Pathology, Medical College of Wisconsin, Milwaukee, Wisconsin, U.S.A.

Thomas P. Lodise, Jr. Albany College of Pharmacy and Health Sciences, Albany, New York, U.S.A.

Linda M. McKinley Department of Infection Control, William S. Middleton Veterans Affairs Medical Center, Madison, Wisconsin, U.S.A.

Isaac Mitropoulos Department of Experimental and Clinical Pharmacology, College of Pharmacy, University of Minnesota, Minneapolis, Minnesota, U.S.A.

Lena M. Napolitano Department of Surgery, University of Michigan Health System, Ann Arbor, Michigan, U.S.A.

Tanyalak Parimon Pulmonary and Critical Care Medicine, Veterans Affairs Medical Center, Boise, Idaho, and Department of Medicine, University of Washington School of Medicine, Seattle, Washington, U.S.A.

R. Lawrence Reed Department of Surgery, Loyola University Medical Center, Maywood, Illinois, U.S.A.

Lee C. Rogers Amputation Prevention Center, Valley Presbyterian Hospital, Los Angeles, California, U.S.A.

John C. Rotschafer Department of Experimental and Clinical Pharmacology, College of Pharmacy, University of Minnesota, Minneapolis, Minnesota, U.S.A.

Nasia Safdar Department of Medicine, University of Wisconsin School of Medicine, University of Wisconsin Hospital and Clinics, and William S. Middleton Veterans Affairs Medical Center, Madison, Wisconsin, U.S.A.

Germana Silva Department of Medicine, University of Wisconsin School of Medicine, University of Wisconsin Hospital and Clinics, and William S. Middleton Veterans Affairs Medical Center, Madison, Wisconsin, U.S.A.

Renae E. Stafford Division of Trauma and Critical Care Surgery, University of North Carolina Department of Surgery

Dennis L. Stevens Infectious Diseases Section, Veterans Affairs Medical Center, Boise, Idaho, and Department of Medicine, University of Washington School of Medicine, Seattle, Washington, U.S.A.

Mary A. Ullman Department of Experimental and Clinical Pharmacology, College of Pharmacy, University of Minnesota, Minneapolis, Minnesota, U.S.A.

John A. Weigelt Department of Surgery, Medical College of Wisconsin, Milwaukee, Wisconsin, U.S.A.

Richard G. Wunderink Division of Pulmonary and Critical Care Medicine, Northwestern University Feinberg School of Medicine, Chicago, Illinois, U.S.A.

Overview of *Staphylococcus aureus* in Medicine

Kent Crossley
Department of Medicine, Veterans Affairs Medical Center, and the University of Minnesota Medical School, Minneapolis, Minnesota, U.S.A.

INTRODUCTION

Staphylococcus aureus has been a major cause of infections in humans for as long as we have historical records. Pathological changes consistent with staphylococcal osteomyelitis are known from Egyptian mummies and other remains of similar antiquity.

Along with several other organisms (e.g., group A β-hemolytic streptococci and *Bacillus anthracis*), this organism is uniquely equipped with virulence factors and defense mechanisms that enable it to cause rapidly progressive fatal infections in normal individuals.

In striking contrast to these bacteria, many organisms that cause health care–associated infections lack well-developed virulence factors and are only able to cause infection because of the absence of normal defenses in the compromised host. Many gram-negative bacteria (e.g., *Pseudomonas* or *Serratia*) and fungi (*Candida* or *Aspergillus* species) rarely cause serious infection in normal individuals. *S. aureus*, almost uniquely among common pathogens, also has an astonishing history of changing clinical manifestations and epidemiological behavior. The sudden appearance of toxic shock syndrome (TSS) 30 years ago and the continuing parallel evolution of antibiotic resistance and virulence are two examples.

COMMUNITY- AND HOSPITAL-ASSOCIATED INFECTION

S. aureus is a major cause of both health care– and community-acquired infections. It is perhaps the single most common cause of hospital-associated infection throughout the world (1). Data are less extensive about community-acquired infection, but it is clear this organism remains an important cause of infection outside of health care settings.

Staphylococci are recognized as common causes of osteomyelitis, skin and soft tissue infection, and bacteremia in normal hosts. Although there are few recent surveys of the causes of community-associated bacteremia, *S. aureus* is a frequent isolate and is associated with significant morbidity and mortality (2,3). Most *S. aureus* infections are minor episodes of cellulitis or cutaneous abscesses. However, serious infections associated with severe systemic toxicity and an abrupt death are not infrequent. Most experienced physicians remember one or more normal young patients who developed bacteremia and endocarditis from a trivial localized infection or who may have developed staphylococcal pneumonia and died in a few days. Rapidly progressive and often fatal infection has been seen in normal young individuals infected with community-acquired methicillin-resistant *S. aureus* (CA-MRSA) infections caused by isolates that contain the Panton–Valentine leukocidin (PVL) (4).

Staphylococcal infection in hospitalized patients has been of major concern for well over a century. Even before the organism was named in the 1880s, clusters of gram-positive cocci had been recognized as the usual cause of suppuration in infected wounds. The gradual introduction of components of "aseptic technique" helped to reduce the frequency of these postoperative infections. The availability of the sulfonamides and penicillins led to a dramatic reduction in the frequency of these infections. By the 1950s, however, prior to the introduction of the semi-synthetic penicillins (e.g., methicillin or oxacillin), penicillin-resistant staphylococci had become a major problem in U.S. hospitals. The introduction of vancomycin and the antistaphylococcal penicillins again brought these infections under control until the arrival of MRSA. Much of the current attention to MRSA is reminiscent of the publicity and anxiety associated with staphylococcal infections in the 1950s.

Thus, long before the recognition of MRSA as a hospital-associated pathogen, *S. aureus* had been a major problem in health care. Examination of National Nosocomial Infections Survey data from the 1980s indicates that *S. aureus* was always one of the most frequent pathogens recovered in hospitals and that it was the most common cause of surgical wound infection (5). It has also been a frequent cause of hospital-associated pneumonia, vascular catheter–associated infection, abscesses, other skin and soft tissue infection, and bacteremia.

METHICILLIN-RESISTANT *STAPHYLOCOCCUS AUREUS*

MRSA was first recognized in the United States in an outbreak reported at Boston City Hospital in the late 1960s (6). These resistant staphylococci were already well established in major European hospitals by that time. For unclear reasons, there were relatively few cases of MRSA infection in the United States until the middle of the following decade. By 1975, outbreaks were being reported with regularity from teaching hospitals and especially from hospitals and units that cared for patients who had been burned (7). Since that time, the frequency of MRSA in hospitalized patients in the United States has continued to grow. Centers for Disease Control and Prevention (CDC) data published in 2007 indicated that most invasive MRSA infections were health care associated and disproportionately distributed; highest incidence rates were in the elderly and in blacks (8).

Although rarely discussed, it is fascinating that MRSA has not replaced more susceptible *S. aureus* as a pathogen (9). Health care institutions have continued to have a baseline number of *S. aureus* hospital-associated infections caused by methicillin-sensitive strains. Infections caused by MRSA are additive to this baseline. Thus, an institution that had 15% of its nosocomial infections caused by *S. aureus* prior to encountering

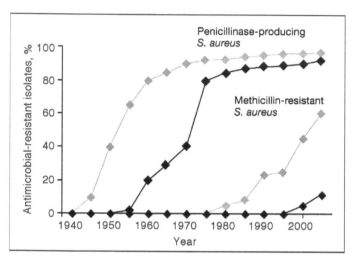

FIGURE 1 Evolution of antimicrobial-resistant *Staphylococcus aureus* as a cause of nosocomial and, then, community-acquired infections. Gray squares represent nosocomial infection and black squares community-acquired infection.

problems with MRSA might, in the following year, have 15% of nosocomial infections caused by sensitive *S. aureus* and an additional 15% caused by MRSA (Fig. 1) (1). This is a major reason that staphylococci are now of so much concern in health care. Not only are these organisms of impressive virulence, they are also more frequent than other causes of nosocomial infection. Nearly 1% of patients discharged from U.S. hospitals in 2000 and 2001 had *S. aureus* infection. These patients were found to have three times the length of hospitalization, three times the total hospital charges, and five times the risk of in-hospital death when compared with inpatients without staphylococcal infection (10).

When staphylococci resistant to penicillin were first seen in the 1950s, they were isolated from patients in hospitals. However, in a relatively few years, these organisms began to replace penicillin-susceptible staphylococci in community-associated infections. A similar process has recently happened with MRSA. Although these isolates were first seen in large acute care hospitals, over the last 10 years they have become frequent causes of typical community-acquired staphylococcal infections. Thus, a patient presenting to an emergency room or urgent care with a carbuncle or infected laceration in 2010 may well have an MRSA isolated even though the patient has not had recent contact with a health care facility (11).

This recent movement of MRSA into the community differs in a major way when compared with the spread of penicillin-resistant staphylococci some 50 years ago. The hospital-associated MRSA have not simply "migrated" into the community. The CA-MRSA are distinct in a variety of ways from the isolates recovered in hospitals. Although the reasons for this are complex, and not entirely understood, it would appear that the genetic determinants of methicillin resistance have been grafted into strains of *S. aureus* that are "epidemiologically virulent." These are organisms that have the necessary virulence factors to be able to cause serious acute infections in normal individuals. They also typically carry other genetic information that specifies antibiotic resistance and allows them to easily spread between individuals and to be effective colonizers. With the addition of the genetic determinant of methicillin resistance (called MecA and carried by a plasmid-like element called the staphylococcus cassette chromosome), strains that are epidemiologically and clinically virulent have become much more problematic for therapy. These CA-MRSA have also been associated with a number of outbreaks of infections in hospitals (12).

EPIDEMIOLOGY OF STAPHYLOCOCCAL INFECTION

Key to understanding how staphylococcal infections develop is an appreciation of the habits of this organism (13). Soon after birth, many neonates become colonized in the anterior nares with *S. aureus*. In adults,

20% to 45% of normal individuals will carry this organism in their anterior nares. It is well recognized that people who frequently use needles, whether for insulin administration, desensitization to allergens, or illicit recreational drug administration, have higher carrier rates than other individuals.

The carrier state is documented to be significantly associated with the development of infections when an injury or skin break occurs (14). A patient known to be nasally colonized with *S. aureus* has a significantly higher risk of developing staphylococcal wound infection after a surgical procedure than someone who is not colonized (15). It is also clear that patients who develop bacteremia with *S. aureus* are usually nasally colonized with the same strain that is recovered from the blood (16). Carriage is a complex topic. Some individuals appear to be chronically colonized; others are only intermittent carriers. Those individuals who are chronically colonized ("persistent carriers") are at highest risk for development of infection following a surgical procedure. In addition to nasal colonization, staphylococci also colonize the peritoneum as well as cutaneous wounds, especially in individuals who are nasal carriers. Although the throat is commonly colonized, the importance of this is not well understood. Carriage is not just a human phenomenon. Household pets may also carry *S. aureus* and have played an important role in some family outbreaks of *S. aureus* disease.

Many individuals who work in hospitals may be nasally colonized. The frequency varies with the extent and type of patient contact. These health care workers often carry the organisms on their fingertips; this is believed to be a consequence of nasal colonization and of hand contamination from other patients and the inanimate environment. Passing of staphylococci between patients through the hands of health care workers is the most frequent way in which these organisms are spread within the health care environment. Prevention of these infections requires careful handwashing on the part of health care workers.

S. *aureus*, like most bacteria, has a variety of structural and enzymatic components that may function in different ways depending on the environment. This enables optimal efficiency for the organism. When there are no antibiotics in the environment, the bacterium has no need to expend energy to maintain antibiotic resistance. The same principle applies to staphylococci as colonizers. Organisms present in the nose are in a semidormant metabolic state. However, once staphylococci reach a site such as a new wound, the organisms have the ability to elaborate a variety of enzymes and toxins that allow them to invade tissues. These same virulence factors are toxic to polymorphonuclear leukocytes and other cells of host defense. Many isolates of S. *aureus* can elaborate a capsule that, as one of its functions, allows the organism to avoid phagocytosis. Once taken up by human leukocytes, staphylococci are able to survive for extended periods and revert to a semidormant state.

CLINICAL INFECTIONS

Skin and Soft Tissue

S. *aureus* may infect any organ or tissue of the body. Infections of the skin, soft tissue, and bone are the most frequent. These infections may range from a localized abscess to more generalized infections such as cellulitis or impetigo. Staphylococcal osteomyelitis is typically the result of a bacteremia in young children, but in older individuals it is related to an adjacent site of infection. Septic bursitis is another common staphylococcal infection. This often involves the olecranon bursa and is almost always caused by S. *aureus*. S. *aureus* is also a frequent cause of vascular catheter–associated infection, postoperative wound infection, and other health care–associated infections.

Although any type of S. *aureus* infection can be associated with the development of TSS, most patients with this illness have infections involving skin and soft tissue. Originally reported as a complication of tampon use in women who had vaginal colonization with S. *aureus*,

TSS is now seen only infrequently. Patients presenting with weakness, postural hypotension, a diffuse pale macular rash, conjunctival injection, and evidence of a localized staphylococcal infection may have TSS.

Bacteremia and Endocarditis

S. aureus accounts for between 15% and 25% of episodes of bacteremia in large-scale studies (2). In individuals who develop their infection in the community, vascular insufficiency and insulin-dependent diabetes are associated with an increased frequency of staphylococcal bacteremia. In hospitalized patients, monitoring devices or vascular catheters are implicated as the source. Mortality in patients with *S. aureus* bacteremia remains between 5% and 30% even with effective antibiotic therapy. Patients with no obvious portal of entry, elderly individuals, and those with serious underlying diseases are at particular risk for death. Identification and management of the source of bacteremia, including early catheter removal, are imperative.

S. aureus is the most frequent cause of acute bacterial endocarditis. It may be acquired in the hospital or community. Most cases are a consequence of an infection acquired as a result of a health care intervention (17). *S. aureus* is capable of causing lethal infection in individuals who do not have preexisting valvular disease. In general, these infections are on the left side of the heart and usually require valve replacement for cure. The use of blood cultures and cardiac ultrasound are usual routes for identifying staphylococcal cardiac infection. Sophisticated clinically derived algorithms are often used to differentiate between uncomplicated bacteremia and the presence of endocarditis (18).

Untreated *S. aureus* bacteremia may be associated with metastatic infection. Patients may develop abscesses involving tissue such as the liver, spleen, or even muscle secondary to bacteremia. Persisting clinical evidence of infections should lead to a methodical search for additional loci of staphylococcal infection in patients who are, or have been, bacteremic.

Pneumonia

S. aureus pneumonia was recognized infrequently in the past and was primarily seen as a complication of influenza. Many of the deaths documented during the 1918 influenza pandemic in young individuals were related to a secondary bacterial superinfection, which was commonly caused by *S. aureus*. In recent years, *S. aureus* isolates that produce the PVL toxin have been associated with skin and soft tissue infection as well as pneumonia in healthy young individuals (19,20). PVL is rapidly cytolytic to white cells. These strains also contain other toxins and virulence factors. This infection is associated with a high mortality rate.

    S. aureus over the years has adapted to new environments and has marshaled resistance to almost all of our available antimicrobial agents. Although vancomycin resistance remains an uncommon issue, MRSA poses a serious treatment challenge at the present time. It seems almost a certainty that, at some point, vancomycin-resistant staphylococci will become the next major treatment challenge mounted by this virulent and adaptable organism.

REFERENCES

1. McDonald LC. Trends in antimicrobial resistance in health care-associated pathogens and effect in treatment. Clin Infect Dis 2006; 42(suppl 2):S65–S71.
2. Shorr AF, Tabak YP, Killian AD, et al. Healthcare associated bloodstream infection: a distinct entity? Insights from a large U.S. database. Crit Care Med 2006; 34(10):2588–2595.
3. Kluytmans-Vandenbergh MF, Kluytmans JA. Community-acquired methicillin-resistant *Staphylococcus aureus*: current perspectives. Clin Microbiol Infect 2006; 12(suppl 1):9–15.
4. Diep BA, Sensabaugh GF, Somboona NS, et al. Widespread skin and soft-tissue infections due to two methicillin-resistant *Staphylococcus aureus* strains harboring the genes for Panton–Valentine leucocidin. J Clin Microbiol 2004; 42:2080–2084.
5. National Nosocomial Infections Surveillance (NNIS) System. A report from the National Nosocomial Infections Surveillance System—data summary

from October 1986–April 1996, issued May 1996. Am J Infect Control 1996; 24:380–388.

6. Barrett FF, McGehee RF Jr., Finland M. Methicillin-resistant *Staphylococcus aureus* at Boston City Hospital. Bacteriologic and epidemiologic observations. N Engl J Med 1968; 279:441–448.

7. Crossley K, Landesman B, Zaske D. An outbreak of infections caused by strains of *Staphylococcus aureus* resistant to methicillin and aminoglycosides. II. Epidemiologic studies. J Infect Dis 1979; 139:280–287.

8. Klevens RM, Morrison MA, Nadle J, et al. Invasive methicillin-resistant *Staphylococcus aureus* infections in the United States. JAMA 2007; 298(15): 1763–1771.

9. Lowy FD. *Staphylococcus aureus* infections. N Engl J Med 1998; 339: 520–532.

10. Noskin GA, Rubin RJ, Schentag JJ, et al. The burden of *Staphylococcus aureus* infections on hospitals in the United States: an analysis of the 2000 and 2001 nationwide inpatient sample database. Arch Intern Med 2005; 165:1756–1761.

11. Moran GJ, Krishnadasan A, Gorwitz RJ, et al. Methicillin-resistant *S. aureus* infections among patients in the emergency department. N Engl J Med 2006; 355:666–674.

12. Seybold U, Kourbatova EV, Johnson JG, et al. Emergence of community-associated methicillin-resistant *Staphylococcus aureus* USA300 genotype as a major cause of health care-associated blood stream infections. Clin Infect Dis 2006; 42:647–56.

13. Wertheim HF, Melles DC, Vos MC, et al. The role of nasal carriage in *Staphylococcus aureus* infections. Lancet Infect Dis 2005; 5:751–762.

14. Safdar N, Bradley EA. The risk of infection after nasal colonization with *Staphylococcus aureus*. Am J Med 2008; 121(4):310–315.

15. Herwaldt LA. *Staphylococcus aureus* nasal carriage and surgical-site infections. Surgery 2003; 134:S2–S9.

16. Von Eiff C, Becker K, Machka K, et al. Nasal carriage as a source of *Staphylococcus aureus* bacteremia. Study Group. N Engl J Med 2001; 344:11–16.

17. Fowler VG Jr., Miro JM, Hoen B, et al. *Staphylococcus aureus* endocarditis: a consequence of medical progress. JAMA 2005; 293:3012–3021.

18. Habib G, Derumeaux G, Avierinos JF, et al. Value and limitations of the Duke criteria for the diagnosis of infective endocarditis. J Am Coll Cardiol 1999; 33:2023–2029.

19. Francis JS, Doherty MC, Lopatin U, et al. Severe community-onset pneumonia in healthy adults caused by methicillin-resistant *Staphylococcus aureus* carrying the Panton–Valentine leukocidin genes. Clin Infect Dis 2005; 40: 100–107.
20. Hidron AI, Low CE, Honig EG, et al. Emergence of community-acquired methicillin-resistant *Staphylococcus aureus* strain USA300 as a cause of necrotizing community-onset pneumonia. Lancet Infect Dis 2009; 9(6): 384–392.

Epidemiology of MRSA

2

Nasia Safdar, Germana Silva, and Barry C. Fox
Department of Medicine, University of Wisconsin School of Medicine,
University of Wisconsin Hospital and Clinics, and William S. Middleton
Veterans Affairs Medical Center, Madison, Wisconsin, U.S.A.

Linda M. McKinley
Department of Infection Control, William S. Middleton Veterans Affairs Medical
Center, Madison, Wisconsin, U.S.A.

INTRODUCTION

Methicillin-resistant *Staphylococcus aureus* (MRSA), a major cause of
infections in healthcare institutions (1) and more recently in the community
(2,3), was first reported in 1961, two years after the introduction of
methicillin for treatment of penicillin-resistant *S. aureus* infections (4,5).
Since then, despite extensive infection control efforts, methicillin resistance
among isolates of *S. aureus* has steadily increased. Data from the National
Healthcare Safety Network (NHSN) at the Centers for Disease Control
and Prevention (CDC) show that 50% to 60% of healthcare–associated
S. aureus isolates from ICUs are now resistant to methicillin. Figure 1
shows resistance trends in *S. aureus* over time (6). Multidrug-resistant
strains of staphylococci are also being reported with increasing frequency
worldwide, including isolates that are resistant to methicillin, lincosamides,
macrolides, aminoglycosides, fluoroquinolones, or combinations of these
antibiotics (7). Recently, the emergence of *S. aureus* strains with intermediate resistance to vancomycin has been reported (8–10). For decades,
vancomycin has been the only uniformly effective treatment against serious
MRSA infections and the development of resistance to it is deeply concerning. MRSA infections are associated with prolonged hospitalization

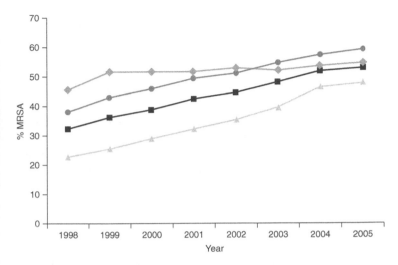

FIGURE 1   MRSA trends (1998–YTD 2005) according to patient location. Data are cumulative: 1998–March 2005. Red line, all patients; yellow line, ICU patients; green line, inpatients; blue line, outpatients. *Abbreviation*: MRSA, methicillin-resistant *Staphylococcus aureus*. *Source*: From Ref. 6.

and increased costs (11,12); some (13,14) but not all (15) studies have reported excess mortality with MRSA infections. Control of spread of MRSA in the healthcare setting and in the community is clearly essential. Understanding the natural history and epidemiology of MRSA colonization and infection is fundamental to devising effective strategies for prevention and control.

COLONIZATION WITH *STAPHYLOCOCCUS AUREUS* AND MRSA

Approximately 30% of the population carry *S. aureus*, usually methicillin-susceptible strains in the nares or on the skin (16). Colonization of the anterior nares with *S. aureus* is a risk factor for invasive infection. A recent study assessed the correlation between strains colonizing the anterior nares and strains in the blood of patients with *S. aureus* bacteremia and found that in 12 of 14 patients the strain causing bacteremia was identical to the strain previously recovered from the anterior nares (17). Determinants of *S. aureus* carriage include host, microbial, and environmental factors.

Studies conducted in acute-care settings show a prevalence of MRSA carriage on admission ranging between 1% and 12% (18–20). As with susceptible strains of *S. aureus*, asymptomatic colonization with MRSA generally precedes infection. In most cases, healthcare–associated infection is a three-step process: (*i*) colonization of the patient's mucosa or skin by a potential pathogen; (*ii*) access of the pathogen to a site where it can invade and produce local infection; and (*iii*) impairment of local host defenses by invasive devices or surgery, fostering invasive infection (21).

Identification of patients likely to be colonized with MRSA on admission is key to promptly deploying contact precautions. Jernigan et al. estimated that the rate of healthcare–associated MRSA transmission was 0.14 transmissions per day and appropriate contact precautions lowered this rate 16-fold (22). A number of risk factors for nosocomial acquisition of MRSA or MRSA carriage on admission to an acute care hospital have been enumerated in several studies. These can be broadly categorized into risk factors intrinsic to the patient such as gender, older age, and comorbidities and extrinsic risk factors such as antimicrobial exposure, use of invasive devices, and the underlying prevalence of MRSA in an institution (23). Interestingly, colonization by methicillin-sensitive *S. aureus* (MSSA) in the nares may protect against establishment of MRSA in that area. Dall et al. tested this hypothesis in a cross-sectional study in patients colonized with MRSA, MSSA, or both and found that colonization by MSSA protected against colonization by MRSA (24).

While the dynamics of MRSA carriage are not entirely understood, it is clear that the risk of invasive infection following colonization with MRSA is greater than the risk of infection following colonization with methicillin-susceptible *S. aureus*. Studies have found that MRSA colonization confers a 3- to 16-fold increased risk for invasive infection compared with MSSA colonization (18,25–27). Patients colonized with MRSA are four times more likely to develop invasive infection than patients colonized with MSSA (Fig. 2) (28).

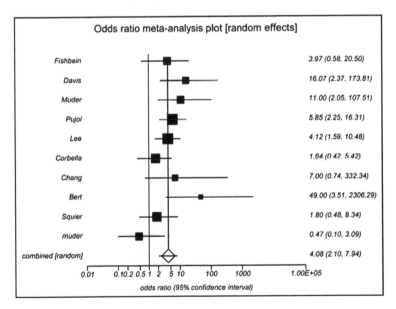

FIGURE 2 Risk of infection after colonization with MRSA compared with the risk of infection after colonization with MSSA. The forest plot shows a fourfold higher risk of infection after colonization with MRSA than MSSA. *Abbreviations*: MRSA, methicillin-resistant *Staphylococcus aureus*; MSSA, methicillin-sensitive *S. aureus*. *Source*: From Ref. 28.

In the community setting, the prevalence of colonization with MRSA is much lower but is thought to be increasing. A recent study using data from the National Health and Nutrition Examination Survey (NHANES) found that the prevalence of colonization with MRSA was 0.84% in the noninstitutionalized U.S. population (29).

Risk Factors for MRSA Carriage at Admission

Variables reflecting prior contact with the healthcare setting are associated with MRSA carriage on admission. A recent study to develop a risk index for predicting patients with MRSA carriage on admission found that the presence of any of the following, age >80 years, previous hospitalization within past 12 months, previous antibiotic use within past six months, and urinary catheter present on admission, would successfully identify the majority of patients with MRSA carriage at admission (30). Prediction rules can identify groups at high risk for carriage with MRSA who may benefit from screening cultures and isolation precautions. In a prospective study of 697 patients, Furuno et al. found that patient self-report of a hospital admission in the previous year had a sensitivity of 76% in identifying patients colonized with MRSA (19). Guidelines from the Society for Healthcare Epidemiology of America recommend screening patients at high risk for MRSA carriage with nasal cultures on admission and periodically throughout hospital stay (31). Contact precautions including the use of a nonsterile gown and gloves prior to entering the patients' room are instituted for patients found to be colonized. Hospitals that have instituted screening recommendations decreased MRSA infection rates (32); nevertheless, costs associated with this approach are substantial and most healthcare institutions do not routinely screen new admissions for MRSA. The ability to accurately predict a high likelihood of MRSA colonization on admission would allow screening cultures for only those patients, thus reducing the cost of this approach.

Risk Factors for Acquisition of Healthcare–Associated MRSA

Among the many risk factors predisposing hospitalized patients to acquiring colonization or developing infection with MRSA, the main modifiable factors are use of invasive devices, colonization pressure, and antimicrobial exposure.

Use of Indwelling Devices

Invasive devices of all types play a far more important role in increasing susceptibility to healthcare–associated infection than underlying diseases. Risk factor analysis shows that most healthcare–associated infections, whether caused by resistant or susceptible microorganisms, derive from invasive procedures or invasive devices. The vast majority of healthcare–associated MRSA bacteremias are intravascular device related. More consistent compliance with evidence-based guidelines for prevention of intravascular device–related bloodstream infection (33,34), ventilator-associated pneumonia (35), surgical site infection (36), and catheter-associated urinary tract infection (37,38), as well as novel technology for preventing device-associated infection (34,38) represent potential strategies for containing MRSA in healthcare institutions. However, translation of evidence into practice is difficult to achieve.

A recent initiative to implement evidence-based guidelines to reduce healthcare–associated device-related infections is found in the Institute for Healthcare Improvement (IHI) 100,000 Lives Campaign, a national initiative with a goal of saving 100,000 lives among patients in hospitals through improvements in healthcare (39). The initiative assembles effective interventions as documented in the peer-reviewed literature into patient care protocols (i.e., care bundles). These care bundles are groupings of best practices with respect to a disease process that individually improve care, but when applied together result in substantially greater improvement than when implemented individually. For example, the central line bundle has five key components: (*i*) hand hygiene, (*ii*) maximal barrier precautions, (*iii*) chlorhexidine skin antisepsis, (*iv*) optimal catheter site selection, with subclavian vein as the preferred site for nontunneled catheters, and (*v*) daily review of line necessity, with prompt removal of unnecessary lines. The approach is most successful when all elements are executed together, an "all or none" strategy.

Colonization Pressure

The prevalence of MRSA colonization or infection in a specific hospital area is a powerful risk factor for individual MRSA acquisition. In a prospective study, Merrer et al. found that weekly colonization pressure (defined as number of MRSA imported + healthcare–associated MRSA patient-days/total no. of patient-days in the week) of 30% or more was associated with a fivefold higher risk of MRSA acquisition (40). Since the major mechanism of healthcare–associated transmission of MRSA is from the hands of healthcare workers, it is plausible that a high colonization pressure, by causing healthcare workers hands to be colonized more frequently, is associated with greater MRSA acquisition. Hand hygiene is fundamental to infection control, and hand hygiene using waterless alcohol–based handrubs reduces nosocomial infections, including those caused by MRSA (41). However, consistent long-term compliance with hand hygiene is difficult to achieve, and many institutions report rates of hand hygiene compliance <50%.

Antimicrobial Exposure

Antimicrobial exposure is another risk factor for the acquisition and transmission of MRSA (42). A number of different classes of antimicrobials are implicated, and both overall institutional use and individual patient use of antimicrobials increase the risk of MRSA. Muller et al. defined the relative contribution of institutional and individual antimicrobial use finding that penicillin use at the hospital level and fluoroquinolone use at the individual level increased the risk of MRSA isolation (43). Other studies found a similar increased risk with fluoroquinolone use (44,45). While the exact mechanism remains unclear, it is likely that the fluoroquinolone effect is mediated by eradication of MSSA and increased expression of adherence factors, both of which may promote colonization by MRSA (46,47). Whether there are differences among the fluoroquinolones as regards the risk of MRSA colonization or infection is unclear. Table 1 summarizes studies that found fluoroquinolone use to be a risk factor for MRSA colonization or infection.

TABLE 1 Fluoroquinolone Exposure as a Risk Factor for MRSA Colonization or Infection

Study	Antimicrobial	Group or individual effect	Estimate of risk
Muller et al. (43)	Penicillins	Group	2.52 (1.15–5.51)
	Fluoroquinolones	Individual	2.63 (1.44–4.80)
Bosso et al. (45)	Fluoroquinolones	Group	Statistically significant increase in MRSA colonization or infection with ciprofloxacin and levofloxacin
Weber et al. (44)	Levofloxacin	Individual	3.38 (1.94–5.90)
	Ciprofloxacin	Individual	2.48 (1.32–4.67)
Graffunder et al. (48)	Levofloxacin	Individual	8.01 (3.15–20.3)
LeBlanc et al. (49)	Fluoroquinolones	Individual	2.57 (1.84–3.60) for colonization and 2.49 (1.02–6.07) for infection

Other antimicrobials such as cephalosporins are also reported to influence the incidence of MRSA. However, most studies have not made a distinction between the effect of an antibiotic at the group level and that at the individual level. Further research is needed to accurately determine the magnitude of risk associated with various antimicrobials for MRSA.

MECHANISMS OF HEALTHCARE–ASSOCIATED TRANSMISSION

Colonized patients are the main reservoir of MRSA. For every patient known to be colonized or infected by multiresistant organisms, a far larger number with unrecognized colonization is already in the institution and, probably, in that patient care unit (50–55). The major mechanism of patient-to-patient spread of resistant microorganisms is on through the hands, equipment, or apparel of healthcare workers (56–62). Of the nurses cultured, 65% showed concordant contamination of their gown or uniform after performing morning care activities for patients with MRSA in urine or a wound (63). Geographic proximity to an infected or colonized patient greatly increases the risk of acquisition of MRSA (59).

Potential Role of the Inanimate Environment

While the role of environmental contamination in contributing to health care–associated infection is unclear, a growing number of studies have found that MRSA may be recovered from hospital equipment and apparatus such as stethoscopes (64), blood pressure cuffs (65), tourniquets (66), and computer terminals (67). The environment is implicated in outbreaks of MRSA that were contained only after environmental cleaning (68,69). Hardy et al. performed serial environmental and patient screening cultures and found that MRSA could be recovered from the environment at every sampling; however, only 3 of 26 patients who acquired MRSA in the hospital acquired it from the environment (70).

Sexton et al. reported that the strains of MRSA causing infection in patients were similar to those recovered from the environment in 70% of patients (71). The CDC guidelines recommend hand hygiene before, in addition to after, patient contact to account for the role of environmental contact transmission (72).

Community-Acquired MRSA

Until recently, MRSA was, with rare exception, a healthcare–associated pathogen. In the last few years, however, multiple studies document cases of MRSA skin and soft tissue infections in the community without traditional risk factors suggesting healthcare–associated MRSA. Termed community-associated or community-acquired MRSA (CA-MRSA), these infections appear to be increasing in incidence. Numerous outbreaks in participants of competitive sports (73), children (74), incarcerated persons (75), military recruits (76), tattoo recipients (77), and more recently, injection drug users (78) and men who have sex with men (64) have been described. Other population groups with high rates of CA-MRSA infections include Alaska natives, native Americans, and Pacific Islanders. The CDC Active Bacterial Core Surveillance Program determined the incidence of endemic CA-MRSA using data from Atlanta, Minnesota, and Baltimore from 2001 through 2002; 1647 cases of community-acquired MRSA infection were reported, representing between 8% and 20% of all MRSA isolates. The annual disease incidence varied according to site and was significantly higher among persons less than two years old than among those who were two years of age or older and among blacks than among whites in Atlanta (79).

CA-MRSA strains, initially only resistant to β-lactams, are becoming more resistant to other antimicrobial agents. The US300 strain is now typically resistant to penicillin, oxacillin, and erythromycin. Variable resistance has been shown to tetracycline and recent isolates have decreased susceptibility to quinolones (80,81).

Differences Between HA-MRSA and CA-MRSA

CA-MRSA is distinct from hospital-acquired MRSA (HA-MRSA) in several ways. Community-associated MRSA is not associated with known risk factors and is much more likely than health care–associated strains to cause skin and soft tissues infections. CA-MRSA strains produce cytotoxins that contribute to inflammation and muscle tissue injury (82). While HA-MRSA strains are typically multidrug resistant, CA-MRSA strains are susceptible to more classes of drugs. Pulsed-field gel electrophoresis (PFGE) typing shows that the US300 strain of *S. aureus* is responsible for much of the CA-MRSA disease burden in the United States (Fig. 3). Outbreaks of CA-MRSA invasive infection in families (84) and in several hospital settings have recently been reported (85).

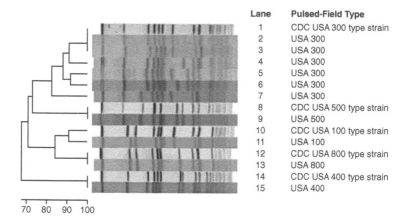

Lane	Pulsed-Field Type
1	CDC USA 300 type strain
2	USA 300
3	USA 300
4	USA 300
5	USA 300
6	USA 300
7	USA 300
8	CDC USA 500 type strain
9	USA 500
10	CDC USA 100 type strain
11	USA 100
12	CDC USA 800 type strain
13	USA 800
14	CDC USA 400 type strain
15	USA 400

70   80   90   100

FIGURE 3 Dendrogram of representative pulsed-field types from MRSA isolates causing skin and soft-tissue infections. The figure shows infections among patients seen at Grady Memorial Hospital (lanes 2 to 7, 9, 11, 13, and 15) and representative MRSA standard-type strains previously published by the CDC (lanes 1, 8, 10, 12, and 14). *Abbreviations*: MRSA, methicillin-resistant *Staphylococcus aureus*; CDC, Centers for Disease Control and Prevention. *Source*: From Ref. 83.

TABLE 2   Characteristics of HA-MRSA and CA-MRSA

Factor	HA-MRSA	CA-MRSA
Risk factors and at risk populations	Previous contact with healthcare settings	Football players, incarcerated persons, military, children
SCC type	Type II	Type IV
PFGE type	US 100	US 300
Toxins	Fewer	More
PVL	Rare	Common
Antibiotic resistance pattern	Multiply resistant	Sensitive to many except β-lactams and erythromycin
Associated clinical syndromes	Bacteremia, pneumonia	Skin and soft tissue infections

Abbreviations: MRSA, methicillin-resistant *Staphylococcus aureus*; HA-MRSA, hospital-acquired MRSA; CA-MRSA, community-acquired MRSA; SCC, staphylococcus cassette chromosome; PFGE, pulsed-field gel electrophoresis; PVL, panton-valentine leucocidin.

Characteristics that are often used to distinguish healthcare–associated MRSA and community-associated MRSA are summarized in Table 2.

REFERENCES

1. Panlilio AL, Culver DH, Gaynes RP, et al. Methicillin-resistant *Staphylococcus aureus* in U.S. hospitals, 1975–1991. Infect Control Hosp Epidemiol 1992; 13(10):582–586.
2. Drews TD, Temte JL, Fox BC. Community-associated methicillin-resistant *Staphylococcus aureus*: review of an emerging public health concern. WMJ 2006; 105(1):52–57.
3. Vandenesch F, Naimi T, Enright MC, et al. Community-acquired methicillin-resistant *Staphylococcus aureus* carrying Panton–Valentine leukocidin genes: worldwide emergence. Emerg Infect Dis 2003; 9(8):978–984.

4. Enright MC, Robinson DA, Randle G, et al. The evolutionary history of methicillin-resistant *Staphylococcus aureus* (MRSA). Proc Natl Acad Sci U S A 2002; 99(11):7687–7692.

5. Jevons MP, Coe AW, Parker MT. Methicillin resistance in staphylococci. Lancet 1963; 1:904–907.

6. Styers D, Sheehan DJ, Hogan P, et al. Laboratory-based surveillance of current antimicrobial resistance patterns and trends among *Staphylococcus aureus*: 2005 status in the United States. Ann Clin Microbiol Antimicrob 2006; 5:2.

7. Deshpande LM, Fritsche TR, Jones RN. Molecular epidemiology of selected multidrug-resistant bacteria: a global report from the SENTRY Antimicrobial Surveillance Program. Diagn Microbiol Infect Dis 2004; 49(4):231–236.

8. Chang S, Sievert DM, Hageman JC, et al. Infection with vancomycin-resistant *Staphylococcus aureus* containing the vanA resistance gene. N Engl J Med 2003; 348(14):1342–1347.

9. Sieradzki K, Roberts RB, Haber SW, et al. The development of vancomycin resistance in a patient with methicillin-resistant *Staphylococcus aureus* infection. N Engl J Med 1999; 340(7):517–523.

10. Smith TL, Pearson ML, Wilcox KR, et al. Emergence of vancomycin resistance in *Staphylococcus aureus*. Glycopeptide-Intermediate *Staphylococcus aureus* Working Group. N Engl J Med 1999; 340(7):493–501.

11. Cosgrove SE, Qi Y, Kaye KS, et al. The impact of methicillin resistance in *Staphylococcus aureus* bacteremia on patient outcomes: mortality, length of stay, and hospital charges. Infect Control Hosp Epidemiol 2005; 26(2):166–174.

12. Engemann JJ, Carmeli Y, Cosgrove SE, et al. Adverse clinical and economic outcomes attributable to methicillin resistance among patients with *Staphylococcus aureus* surgical site infection. Clin Infect Dis 2003; 36(5):592–598.

13. Chang FY, MacDonald BB, Peacock JE Jr., et al. A prospective multicenter study of *Staphylococcus aureus* bacteremia: incidence of endocarditis, risk factors for mortality, and clinical impact of methicillin resistance. Medicine (Baltimore) 2003; 82(5):322–332.

14. Ridenour GA, Wong ES, Call MA, et al. Duration of colonization with methicillin-resistant *Staphylococcus aureus* among patients in the intensive care unit: implications for intervention. Infect Control Hosp Epidemiol 2006; 27(3):271–278.

15. Zahar JR, Clec'h C, Tafflet M, et al. Is methicillin resistance associated with a worse prognosis in *Staphylococcus aureus* ventilator-associated pneumonia? Clin Infect Dis 2005; 41(9):1224–1231.

16. Wertheim HF, Melles DC, Vos MC, et al. The role of nasal carriage in *Staphylococcus aureus* infections. Lancet Infect Dis 2005; 5(12):751–762.

17. von Eiff C, Becker K, Machka K, et al. Nasal carriage as a source of *Staphylococcus aureus* bacteremia. Study Group. N Engl J Med 2001; 344(1): 11–16.

18. Cutler CJ, Davis N. Improving oral care in patients receiving mechanical ventilation. Am J Crit Care 2005; 14(5):389–394.

19. Furuno JP, Harris AD, Wright MO, et al. Prediction rules to identify patients with methicillin-resistant *Staphylococcus aureus* and vancomycin-resistant enterococci upon hospital admission. Am J Infect Control 2004; 32(8): 436–440.

20. Samad A, Banerjee D, Carbarns N, et al. Prevalence of methicillin-resistant *Staphylococcus aureus* colonization in surgical patients, on admission to a Welsh hospital. J Hosp Infect 2002; 51(1):43–46.

21. Bonten MJ, Bergmans DC, Ambergen AW, et al. Risk factors for pneumonia, and colonization of respiratory tract and stomach in mechanically ventilated ICU patients. Am J Respir Crit Care Med 1996; 154(5):1339–1346.

22. Jernigan JA, Titus MG, Groschel DH, et al. Effectiveness of contact isolation during a hospital outbreak of methicillin-resistant *Staphylococcus aureus*. Am J Epidemiol 1996; 143(5):496–504.

23. Safdar N, Maki DG. The commonality of risk factors for nosocomial colonization and infection with antimicrobial-resistant *Staphylococcus aureus*, *Enterococcus*, gram-negative bacilli, *Clostridium difficile*, and *Candida*. Ann Intern Med 2002; 136(11):834–844.

24. Dall'Antonia M, Coen PG, Wilks M, et al. Competition between methicillin-sensitive and -resistant *Staphylococcus aureus* in the anterior nares. J Hosp Infect 2005; 61(1):62–67.

25. Fishbain JT, Lee JC, Nguyen HD, et al. Nosocomial transmission of methicillin-resistant *Staphylococcus aureus*: a blinded study to establish baseline acquisition rates. Infect Control Hosp Epidemiol 2003; 24(6): 415–421.

26. Pujol M, Pena C, Pallares R, et al. Nosocomial *Staphylococcus aureus* bacteremia among nasal carriers of methicillin-resistant and methicillin-susceptible strains. Am J Med 1996; 100(5):509–516.

27. Muder RR, Brennen C, Wagener MM, et al. Methicillin-resistant staphylococcal colonization and infection in a long-term care facility. Ann Intern Med 1991; 114(2):107–112.

28. Safdar N, Bradley EA. The risk of infection after nasal colonization with *Staphylococcus aureus*. Am J Med 2008; 121(4):310–315.
29. Graham PL, III, Lin SX, Larson EL. A U.S. population-based survey of *Staphylococcus aureus* colonization. Ann Intern Med 2006; 144(5):318–325.
30. Harbarth S, Sax H, Fankhauser-Rodriguez C, et al. Evaluating the probability of previously unknown carriage of MRSA at hospital admission. Am J Med 2006; 119(3):275.e15–e23.
31. Muto CA, Jernigan JA, Ostrowsky BE, et al. SHEA guideline for preventing nosocomial transmission of multidrug-resistant strains of *Staphylococcus aureus* and *Enterococcus*. Infect Control Hosp Epidemiol 2003; 24(5):362–386.
32. Bonuel N, Byers P, Gray-Becknell T. Methicillin resistant *Staphylococcus aureus* (MRSA) prevention through facility-wide culture change. Crit Care Nurs Q 2009; 32(2):144–148.
33. O'Grady NP, Alexander M, Dellinger EP, et al. Guidelines for the prevention of intravascular catheter-related infections. Centers for Disease Control and Prevention. MMWR Recomm Rep 2002; 51(RR-10):1–29.
34. Safdar N, Crnich CJ, Maki DG. The pathogenesis of ventilator-associated pneumonia: its relevance to developing effective strategies for prevention. Respir Care 2005; 50(6):725–739; discussion 739–741.
35. Tablan OC, Anderson LJ, Besser R, et al. Guidelines for preventing health-care–associated pneumonia, 2003: recommendations of CDC and the healthcare infection control practices advisory committee. MMWR Recomm Rep 2004; 53(RR-3):1–36.
36. Mangram AJ, Horan TC, Pearson ML, et al. Guideline for prevention of surgical site infection, 1999. Centers for Disease Control and Prevention (CDC) Hospital Infection Control Practices Advisory Committee. Am J Infect Control 1999; 27(2):97–132; quiz 133–134; discussion 96.
37. Climo M, Diekema D, Warren DK, et al. Prevalence of the use of central venous access devices within and outside of the intensive care unit: results of a survey among hospitals in the prevention epicenter program of the Centers for Disease Control and Prevention. Infect Control Hosp Epidemiol 2003; 24(12):942–945.
38. Maki DG, Tambyah PA. Engineering out the risk for infection with urinary catheters. Emerg Infect Dis 2001; 7(2):342–347.
39. Berwick DM, Calkins DR, McCannon CJ, et al. The 100,000 lives campaign: setting a goal and a deadline for improving health care quality. JAMA 2006; 295(3):324–327.

40. Merrer J, Santoli F, Appere de Vecchi C, et al. "Colonization pressure" and risk of acquisition of methicillin-resistant *Staphylococcus aureus* in a medical intensive care unit. Infect Control Hosp Epidemiol 2000; 21(11):718–723.

41. Pittet D, Hugonnet S, Harbarth S, et al. Effectiveness of a hospital-wide programme to improve compliance with hand hygiene. Infection Control Programme. Lancet 2000; 356(9238):1307–1312.

42. Muller AA, Mauny F, Bertin M, et al. Relationship between spread of methicillin-resistant *Staphylococcus aureus* and antimicrobial use in a French university hospital. Clin Infect Dis 2003; 36(8):971–978.

43. Muller A, Mauny F, Talon D, et al. Effect of individual- and group-level antibiotic exposure on MRSA isolation: a multilevel analysis. J Antimicrob Chemother 2006; 58(4):878–881.

44. Weber SG, Gold HS, Hooper DC, et al. Fluoroquinolones and the risk for methicillin-resistant *Staphylococcus aureus* in hospitalized patients. Emerg Infect Dis 2003; 9(11):1415–1422.

45. Bosso JA, Mauldin PD. Using interrupted time series analysis to assess associations of fluoroquinolone formulary changes with susceptibility of gram-negative pathogens and isolation rates of methicillin-resistant *Staphylococcus aureus*. Antimicrob Agents Chemother 2006; 50(6):2106–2112.

46. Bisognano C, Vaudaux P, Rohner P, et al. Induction of fibronectin-binding proteins and increased adhesion of quinolone-resistant *Staphylococcus aureus* by subinhibitory levels of ciprofloxacin. Antimicrob Agents Chemother 2000; 44(6):1428–1437.

47. Bisognano C, Vaudaux PE, Lew DP, et al. Increased expression of fibronectin-binding proteins by fluoroquinolone-resistant *Staphylococcus aureus* exposed to subinhibitory levels of ciprofloxacin. Antimicrob Agents Chemother 1997; 41(5):906–913.

48. Graffunder EM, Venezia RA. Risk factors associated with nosocomial methicillin-resistant *Staphylococcus aureus* (MRSA) infection including previous use of antimicrobials. J Antimicrob Chemother 2002; 49(6):999–1005.

49. LeBlanc L, Pepin J, Toulouse K, et al. Fluoroquinolones and risk for methicillin-resistant *Staphylococcus aureus*, Canada. Emerg Infect Dis 2006; 12(9):1398–1405.

50. Martone WJ. Spread of vancomycin-resistant enterococci: why did it happen in the United States? Infect Control Hosp Epidemiol 1998; 19:539–545.

51. Tucci V, Haran MA, Isenberg HD. Epidemiology and control of vancomycin-resistant enterococci in an adult and children's hospital. Am J Infect Control 1997; 25:371–376.

52. Yokoe DS, Mermel LA, Anderson DJ, et al. A compendium of strategies to prevent healthcare-associated infections in acute care hospitals. Infect Control Hosp Epidemiol 2008; 29(suppl 1):S12–S21.

53. Boyce JM, Opal SM, Chow JW, et al. Outbreak of multidrug-resistant *Enterococcus faecium* with transferable vanB class vancomycin resistance. J Clin Microbiol 1994; 32(5):1148–1153.

54. Montecalvo MA, Jarvis WR, Uman J, et al. Infection-control measures reduce transmission of vancomycin-resistant enterococci in an endemic setting. Ann Int Med 1999; 131(4):269–272.

55. Quale J, Landman D, Atwood E, et al. Experience with a hospital-wide outbreak of vancomycin-resistant enterococci. Am J Infect Control 1996; 24(5):372–379.

56. Knittle MA, Eitzman DV, Baer H. Role of hand contamination of personnel in the epidemiology of gram-negative nosocomial infections. J Pediatr 1975; 86(3):433–437.

57. Handwerger S, Raucher B, Altarac D, et al. Nosocomial outbreak due to *Enterococcus faecium* highly resistant to vancomycin, penicillin, and gentamicin. Clin Infect Dis 1993; 16(6):750–755.

58. Zachary KC, Bayne PS, Morrison VJ, et al. Contamination of gowns, gloves, and stethoscopes with vancomycin-resistant enterococci. Infect Control Hosp Epidemiol 2001; 22:560–564.

59. Peacock JE Jr., Marsik FJ, Wenzel RP. Methicillin-resistant *Staphylococcus aureus*: introduction and spread within a hospital. Ann Intern Med 1980; 93(4):526–532.

60. Thompson RL, Cabezudo I, Wenzel RP. Epidemiology of nosocomial infections caused by methicillin-resistant *Staphylococcus aureus*. Ann Intern Med 1982; 97(3):309–317.

61. Crossley K, Landesman B, Zaske D. An outbreak of infections caused by strains of *Staphylococcus aureus* resistant to methicillin and aminoglycosides. II. Epidemiologic studies. J Infect Dis 1979; 139(3):280–287.

62. Crossley K, Loesch D, Landesman B, et al. An outbreak of infections caused by strains of *Staphylococcus aureus* resistant to methicillin and aminoglycosides. I. Clinical studies. J Infect Dis 1979; 139(3):273–279.

63. Boyce JM, Chenevert C. Isolation gowns prevent health care workers (HCWs) from contaminating their clothing, and possibly their hands, with methicillin-resistant *Staphylococcus aureus* (MRSA) and resistant enterococci. The Eighth Annual Meeting of the Society for Healthcare Epidemiology of America. Orlando, FL, 1998:72.

64. Szumowski JD, Wener KM, Gold HS, et al. Methicillin-resistant *Staphylococcus aureus* colonization, behavioral risk factors, and skin and soft-tissue infection at an ambulatory clinic serving a large population of HIV-infected men who have sex with men. Clin Infect Dis 2009; 49(1):118–121.
65. Layton MC, Perez M, Heald P, et al. An outbreak of mupirocin-resistant *Staphylococcus aureus* on a dermatology ward associated with an environmental reservoir. Infect Control Hosp Epidemiol 1993; 14(7):369–375.
66. Berman DS, Schaefler S, Simberkoff MS, et al. Tourniquets and nosocomial methicillin-resistant *Staphylococcus aureus* infections. N Engl J Med 1986; 315(8):514–515.
67. Devine J, Cooke RP, Wright EP. Is methicillin-resistant *Staphylococcus aureus* (MRSA) contamination of ward-based computer terminals a surrogate marker for nosocomial MRSA transmission and handwashing compliance? J Hosp Infect 2001; 48(1):72–75.
68. Embil JM, McLeod JA, Al-Barrak AM, et al. An outbreak of methicillin resistant *Staphylococcus aureus* on a burn unit: potential role of contaminated hydrotherapy equipment. Burns 2001; 27(7):681–688.
69. Kumari DN, Haji TC, Keer V, et al. Ventilation grilles as a potential source of methicillin-resistant *Staphylococcus aureus* causing an outbreak in an orthopaedic ward at a district general hospital. J Hosp Infect 1998; 39(2): 127–133.
70. Hardy KJ, Oppenheim BA, Gossain S, et al. A study of the relationship between environmental contamination with methicillin-resistant *Staphylococcus aureus* (MRSA) and patients' acquisition of MRSA. Infect Control Hosp Epidemiol 2006; 27(2):127–132.
71. Sexton T, Clarke P, O'Neill E, et al. Environmental reservoirs of methicillin-resistant *Staphylococcus aureus* in isolation rooms: correlation with patient isolates and implications for hospital hygiene. J Hosp Infect 2006; 62(2): 187–194.
72. Boyce JM, Pittet D. Guideline for hand hygiene in health-care settings. Recommendations of the healthcare infection control practices advisory committee and the HICPAC/SHEA/APIC/IDSA hand hygiene task force. Society for Healthcare Epidemiology of America/Association for Professionals in Infection Control/Infectious Diseases Society of America. MMWR Recomm Rep 2002; 51(RR-16):1–45, quiz CE 1–4.
73. Kazakova SV, Hageman JC, Matava M, et al. A clone of methicillin-resistant *Staphylococcus aureus* among professional football players. N Engl J Med 2005; 352(5):468–475.

74. Herold BC, Immergluck LC, Maranan MC, et al. Community-acquired methicillin-resistant *Staphylococcus aureus* in children with no identified predisposing risk. JAMA 1998; 279(8):593–598.

75. Methicillin-resistant *Staphylococcus aureus* infections in correctional facilities—Georgia, California, and Texas, 2001–2003. MMWR Morb Mortal Wkly Rep 2003; 52(41):992–996.

76. Campbell KM, Vaughn AF, Russell KL, et al. Risk factors for community-associated methicillin-resistant *Staphylococcus aureus* infections in an outbreak of disease among military trainees in San Diego, California, in 2002. J Clin Microbiol 2004; 42(9):4050–4053.

77. Dillman DA. Why choice of survey mode makes a difference. Public Health Rep 2006; 121(1):11–13.

78. Atkinson SR, Paul J, Sloan E, et al. The emergence of methicillin-resistant *Staphylococcus aureus* among injecting drug users. J Infect 2009; 58(5):339–345.

79. Fridkin SK, Hageman JC, Morrison M, et al. Methicillin-resistant *Staphylococcus aureus* disease in three communities. N Engl J Med 2005; 352(14): 1436–1444.

80. Como-Sabetti K, Harriman KH, Buck JM, et al. Community-associated methicillin-resistant *Staphylococcus aureus*: trends in case and isolate characteristics from six years of prospective surveillance. Public Health Rep 2009; 124(3):427–435.

81. Tenover FC, McDougal LK, Goering RV, et al. Characterization of a strain of community-associated methicillin-resistant *Staphylococcus aureus* widely disseminated in the United States. J Clin Microbiol 2006; 44(1):108–118.

82. Tseng CW, Kyme P, Low J, et al. *Staphylococcus aureus* Panton–Valentine leukocidin contributes to inflammation and muscle tissue injury. PLoS One 2009; 4(7):e6387.

83. King MD, Humphrey BJ, Wang YF, et al. Emergence of community-acquired methicillin-resistant *Staphylococcus aureus* USA300 clone as the predominant cause of skin and soft-tissue infections. Ann Intern Med 2006; 144(5): 309–317.

84. Huijsdens XW, van Santen-Verheuvel MG, Spalburg E, et al. Multiple cases of familial transmission of community-acquired methicillin-resistant *Staphylococcus aureus*. J Clin Microbiol 2006; 44(8):2994–2996.

85. Jenkins TC, McCollister BD, Sharma R, et al. Epidemiology of healthcare-associated bloodstream infection caused by USA300 strains of methicillin-resistant *Staphylococcus aureus* in 3 affiliated hospitals. Infect Control Hosp Epidemiol 2009; 30(3):233–241.

MRSA: Genetics, Virulence Factors, and Toxin Expression

Dennis L. Stevens
Infectious Diseases Section, Veterans Affairs Medical Center, Boise, Idaho,
and Department of Medicine, University of Washington School of Medicine,
Seattle, Washington, U.S.A.

Tanyalak Parimon
Pulmonary and Critical Care Medicine, Veterans Affairs Medical Center, Boise,
Idaho, and Department of Medicine, University of Washington School of
Medicine, Seattle, Washington, U.S.A.

Amy E. Bryant
Infectious Diseases Section, Veterans Affairs Medical Center, Boise, Idaho,
and Department of Medicine, University of Washington School of Medicine,
Seattle, Washington, U.S.A.

INTRODUCTION

Staphylococcus aureus is once again reemerging as a major threat to
human health and well-being the world over. As humans and medicine
have evolved, *S. aureus* too has evolved and adapted to a wide variety of
human conditions and medical innovations. Historically, *S. aureus* was
certainly a significant human pathogen prior to the development of antibiotics. For example, in the last century, *S. aureus* was a major bacterial
cause of death in the influenza pandemic of 1918 among those who
developed secondary bacterial pneumonia. Following the introduction of
antibiotics in the 1940s, *S. aureus* developed resistance to penicillin, and
then emerged as an important cause of serious nosocomial infections in the
1950s. With the development and widespread use of chloramphenicol and

tetracycline in the 1960s, superinfections due to *S. aureus* occurred including staphylococcal enterocolitis. These were clearly related to two factors: antibiotic eradication of the normal gut flora and concomitant proliferation of *S. aureus* strains that had developed antibiotic resistance during treatment. The timely discovery of β-lactamase-resistant cephalosporins and later the semisynthetic β-lactam antibiotics (methicillin, oxacillin, and nafcillin) saved the day for the next 10 to 15 years. Still, as early as the 1970s, sporadic reports of methicillin-resistant *S. aureus* (MRSA) began to appear. Epidemics of MRSA were reported in some unique facilities with extremely ill patients and with intense antibiotic usage (1). Over the subsequent 20 to 30 years, we have seen the widespread emergence of MRSA infections in certain regions of Europe, throughout the United States, as well as in Japan and the Western Pacific. Until very recently, these MRSA strains have largely been associated with hospital-acquired infections (HA-MRSA) (2,3).

COMMUNITY-ACQUIRED MRSA: GENETIC DIFFERENCES

Only recently have reports of true community-acquired MRSA (CA-MRSA) infections begun to emerge (4–6). Empiric treatment of some of these with conventional agents was inadequate and resulted in disastrous outcomes before it was determined that the etiologic agent was MRSA (7). There are two lessons to be learned from these dramatic cases. First, these infections did not respond to the types of agents that most physicians would prescribe for community-acquired *S. aureus* infections. Second, these were particularly severe types of infections as they resulted in deaths. Thus, these CA-MRSA strains were unique not only because of methicillin resistance, but also because they were highly virulent. Epidemiologic studies using molecular tools are rapidly replacing classical epidemiology and have provided great insight into the pathogenesis of these infections. For instance, the classical studies concluded that patients with CA-MRSA infection in these early reports must have had some type of contact with health care facilities, occult antibiotic exposure, or contact with someone with HA-MRSA. However, pulsed field gel electrophoresis comparing strains from the community and those from hospital-associated infection demonstrated that multiple different strains were causing the hospital-associated infections, whereas there was an identical pattern for CA-MRSA causing diverse infections from widely disparate geographical areas (8), suggesting a clonal distribution of a unique community-associated *S. aureus* strain now designated USA300.

Indeed, there is now clear genetic-based evidence that CA-MRSA strains are distinct from HA-MRSA (8,9). In fact, Daum et al. (9) demonstrated that there are at least four different types of *mecA* (methicillin resistance) gene cassettes. Interestingly, type I, II, and III are associated with strains causing HA-MRSA infections, whereas type IV distinguishes CA-MRSA infections. The type IV *mecA* gene cassette is much smaller (23 kDa) compared to types I, II, and III that are 95, 80, and 55 kDa, respectively. If smaller size is in fact associated with a greater likelihood of transfer to sensitive strains, then many strains of *S. aureus* in the community could acquire *mecA* gene cassette type IV and the prevalence of CA-MRSA infections should increase dramatically. Indeed, this phenomenon has come to fruition, and recent estimates document that 59% of staphylococcal species causing skin and soft tissue infections in the outpatient setting are in fact CA-MRSA (10).

Additional reports document an increasing frequency of CA-MRSA infections in the pediatric population (4–7). On the basis of the striking similarity in the patterns of the USA300 strains of CA-MRSA, these have been referred to as a clone. It seems likely that the origin of USA300 was a methicillin-sensitive *S. aureus* (MSSA) strain, probably phage type 80/81, which acquired the type IV *mecA* gene. In fact, with more refined genetic analysis, new evidence suggests there are many different MSSA strains that have acquired the type IV *mecA* gene (Robert Daum, personal communication). Thus, there are likely multiple unique strains of CA-MRSA throughout the United States.

Unique Syndromes Caused by Toxin-Producing Strains of *Staphylococcus aureus*

Although the adaptability of *S. aureus* to antibiotics is well documented, the acquisition and expression of virulence genes has not been extensively studied. Still, we are well aware historically of the emergence of novel clinical syndromes such as staphylococcal scalded skin syndrome (SSSS), staphylococcal toxic shock syndrome (StaphTSS), staphylococcal food poisoning, and more recently necrotizing fasciitis (11) and hemorrhagic necrotizing pneumonia (12). In each case, these novel syndromes have been the result of acquiring mobile genetic elements, usually via bacteriophage, with subsequent expression of specific extracellular toxins.

Staphylococcus aureus: Genetic Elements, Surface Components, and Extracellular Toxins

To understand the complexity of MRSA colonization and infection at the present time, it is important to have a perspective on the genetics, surface structures, metabolism, and extracellular virulence factors of *S. aureus* that contribute to pathogenesis.

Staphylococci are nonsporulating, nonmotile gram-positive cocci that have an average diameter of 1 mm and microscopically appear as grapelike clusters. When grown on blood agar, staphylococci form small (1–2 mm), smooth, round colonies that are often yellow pigmented and may be surrounded by a zone of β-hemolysis. Staphylococci are very hardy organisms and can withstand much more physical and chemical stress than pneumococci and streptococci. For example, staphylococci resist drying, withstand 10% NaCl, and will survive and even replicate at temperatures between 10°C and 45°C. Because staphylococci are facultative anaerobes, they will grow with or without oxygen.

The cellular structure of *S. aureus* is complex and most strains have polysaccharide microcapsules. The cell wall of *S. aureus* is structurally similar to that of group A streptococcus in that both have a carbohydrate antigen, a protein component, and a mucopeptide. The carbohydrate antigen is a teichoic acid, which in *S. aureus* is a polymer of *N*-acetylglucosamine and polyribitol phosphate. Antibodies to teichoic acid can be detected in normal human serum, and elevated antibody titers are present in patients with deep-seated staphylococcal infections. Teichoic acid has no established role in virulence, and antibodies to this carbohydrate are not protective. The protein component of the cell wall includes protein A, which binds IgG from multiple species including humans (13). Protein A interacts with the Fc component of IgG (as opposed to the Fab region) and hence it is not a true antigen. Protein A may be antiphagocytic, but its role in virulence has not been clearly established. The staphylococcal cell wall mucopeptide is structurally similar to the mucopeptide of other gram-positive bacteria.

Most strains of *S. aureus* produce a variety of extracellular products, including both enzymes and toxins that may account for the tendency to produce burrowing, destructive, localized infections. The enzyme coagulase causes plasma to clot, thus promoting the fibrin meshwork that contributes to abscess formation. Staphylococci can also produce lipase, protease, hyaluronidase, and DNAse—each of which can add to tissue damage. Another important enzyme is penicillinase. Because penicillinase has no role in pathogenicity, staphylococci that produce this enzyme are no more virulent than non-penicillinase-producing strains. Nevertheless, this enzyme is clinically and epidemiologically important because it hydrolyzes the β-lactam ring of penicillin, thereby inactivating the molecule. The production of penicillinase is controlled by plasmids, or episomes, that are extrachromosomal DNA molecules that replicate during cell division. Unlike the R factors of gram-negative bacilli, the plasmids responsible for penicillinase production do not usually mediate resistance to multiple antibiotics.

Of even greater interest are the non-enzymatic exotoxins produced by *S. aureus*. α-Toxin (also known as α-hemolysin), encoded by the *hla* gene, is a pore-forming cytotoxin that alters host cell membrane permeability and results in cell damage or death. α-Toxin injures red and white blood cells, and epithelial and endothelial cells. It also activates platelets.

Injection of α-toxin into animals can produce dermal necrosis and contraction of vascular smooth muscle, leading to tissue ischemia. In experimental studies, α-toxin stimulated apoptosis of endothelial cells causing vascular injury (14) as well as necrosis of respiratory and alveolar epithelial cells, resulting in pulmonary edema and acute lung injury (15). In a murine pneumonia model, isogenic *hla*-deficient mutants of *S. aureus* demonstrated reduced virulence compared with the wild-type parent strain (16–18). Fewer neutrophils infiltrated lung tissue in mice infected with the *hla*-deficient strain because of reduced secretion of neutrophil chemoattractants in the airway, suggesting that α-toxin promotes neutrophil-dependent destruction of lung tissue (18). Future studies will fully elucidate the mechanisms by which α-toxin contributes to staphylococcal disease.

S. aureus also produces a family of bi-component leukocidins that disrupt plasma and lysosomal membranes of neutrophils, monocytes, and macrophages, resulting in degranulation, inflammatory mediator release, and cell apoptosis (19). Recently, the Panton–Valentine leukocidin (PVL), encoded by the genes *lukS*-PV and *lukF*-PV, has gained renewed attention, having been epidemiologically linked to cases of CA-MRSA infections (20–23), though controversy remains regarding its role in pathogenesis (24–26). Although the prevalence of PVL is enriched in strains associated with certain categories of severe community-acquired infection [e.g., hemorrhagic or necrotizing pneumonia, 100% (12); necrotizing fasciitis, 100% (11); and pyomyositis, 100% (27)], most strains causing simple abscesses, carbuncles, and furuncles also have the PVL genes (28). We have shown that no direct correlation exists between the amount of PVL produced in vitro and the severity of infection (29). In fact, the highest PVL producers were strains isolated from abscesses whereas strains isolated from patients with hemorrhagic/necrotizing pneumonia or necrotizing fasciitis were only moderate producers of PVL (29). Thus, there has not been a clear causal relationship of PVL to severe infection.

StaphTSS caused by MRSA has been reported in numerous studies (9,30–35). In the past, StaphTSS has been caused by toxic shock syndrome toxin-1 (TSST-1)-producing strains isolated from patients with tampon-associated menstrual cases and by staphylococcal enterotoxin B (SEB)-producing strains isolated from post-surgical cases associated with wound-packing material. The gene TSST-1 has rarely been found in CA-MRSA, and virtually never in conjunction with the genes for PVL (Perdreau-Remington, personal communication). In 2007, however, among blood isolates from Holland, the TSST-1 gene was found in 3% of MRSA and 11% of MSSA (34) suggesting that StaphTSS might become more common and manifest itself in a variety of new situations.

Occasionally, strains of staphylococci produce exfoliatin that causes the epidermolysis of staphylococcal scalded skin syndrome. Some strains of staphylococci can also produce one of four antigenically distinct enterotoxins that cause the vomiting and diarrhea characteristic of staphylococcal food poisoning. In rare instances, staphylococci produce an erythrogenic toxin that causes scarlet fever.

Pathogenesis of Staphylococcal Infections

The earliest tissue response in staphylococcal infection is acute inflammation with a vigorous exudation of polymorphonuclear leukocytes. Vascular thrombosis and tissue necrosis quickly lead to abscess formation. As a result of the development of a fibrin meshwork and later fibroblast proliferation, these abscesses become walled-off zones of loculated infection and tissue destruction, with dying leukocytes and viable bacteria at the center. Fibrosis and scarring are often prominent in healing.

The importance of the granulocyte in host defense is supported by the enhanced susceptibility to staphylococcal infections seen in patients with neutropenia or various disorders of neutrophil function, such as chronic granulomatous disease, Chédiak–Higashi syndrome, and various disorders of chemotaxis. The most important factors predisposing to staphylococcal infections are not immunologic defects but mechanical defects. Minute skin abrasions, for example, probably provide the portal of entry in staphylococcal skin infections and in many cases of staphylococcal bacteremia. Intravenous drug abuse accounts for many cases of staphylococcal bacteremia and endocarditis. Indwelling venous catheters are particularly important in nosocomial infections; plastic catheters become coated with fibrinogen and fibrin, which interact with adhesions on the bacterial cell surface and bind staphylococci to the catheter.

ARE COMMUNITY-ACQUIRED-MRSA STRAINS MORE VIRULENT?

A major concern is the increased potential for more serious CA-MRSA infections. Some investigations have demonstrated a two-fold increase in the prevalence of TSST-1 and staphylococcal enterotoxin in MRSA strains compared with MSSA strains (11). In fact, recent reports from Japan suggest an increase in the frequency of StaphTSS caused by MRSA (12,13,20). In addition, the propensity of MRSA to cause more severe soft tissue infections is suggested by the fatal cases recently reported from the Midwest of the United States (6), by the reports of necrotizing fasciitis caused by CA-MRSA and by fulminant necrotizing hemorrhagic pneumonia following influenza. Similarly, severe staphylococcal infections in France have been reported to be associated with the Panton–Valentine leukocidin (23,31,36–38). Recent studies in the United States have shown that this toxin is found in 77% of CA-MRSA strains compared with 14% of HA-MRSA and 0% of methicillin-sensitive strains (39), including bacteremia, pneumonia, and soft tissue infections. In the future, StaphTSS may not be limited to menstrual cases or post-surgical cases involving packing material. In addition, pneumonia may be more severe based on recent studies in France (21–23). Finally, necrotizing soft tissue infections may become more common because of the presence of the Panton–Valentine leukocidin (21–23).

THE EMPIRIC CHOICE OF ANTIMICROBIAL TREATMENT

Clearly, we have learned lessons from patients with HA-MRSA. When the prevalence of MRSA in our hospitals increased from 0% to 30–40%, empiric treatment of staphylococcal infection demanded administration of agents such as vancomycin to which the organism remained sensitive. Selection of an effective antibiotic regimen also required that clinicians be supplied with the most up-to-date information regarding the prevalence of MRSA in their specific hospitals. However, if we are to adequately treat emerging CA-MRSA infections, we must also know the prevalence of MRSA strains in our community. Clearly, this will require that CA-MRSA infections become reportable. At the bedside, in evaluating patients with community-acquired staphylococcal infection who are seriously ill, we cannot assume that nafcillin or a cephalosporin will be an effective treatment. Thus, the two most important factors guiding antibiotic treatment in this setting will be the prevalence of MRSA in our area and the severity of the illness. Particularly with seriously ill patients, it will be prudent to assume that the infection is caused by MRSA and begin empiric treatment with agents effective against MRSA. As alluded to previously, there are genetic reasons to suspect that MRSA strains may turn out to be more virulent, but this notion will need to be proven by good epidemiologic studies. In less seriously ill patients, conventional treatment may be sufficient, but we must recognize that such therapy may fail, and careful clinical follow-up will be necessary. More than ever, making a correct diagnosis and obtaining good culture material for susceptibility testing will be crucial for rational antibiotic selection and switching. Should CA-MRSA strains be isolated, careful follow-up, monitoring of the patients' clinical course, and changing therapy promptly will be necessary to ensure good outcomes.

SPECIFIC CONSIDERATIONS IN THE SELECTION OF SPECIFIC ANTI-MRSA ANTIMICROBIAL AGENTS

Skin and Soft Tissue Infections

Numerous clinical trials have documented the efficacy of linezolid, vancomycin, daptomycin, and glycycline in skin and soft tissue infections (39,40).

Pneumonia

There may be some advantage for linezolid because of its excellent penetration into lung alveolar fluid (41). Daptomycin should not be used to treat bacterial pneumonia because of its high protein binding and inactivation by surfactant. Tigecycline has not yet been studied in the treatment of pneumonia.

Bacteremia and Endocarditis

Linezolid and vancomycin are equivalent in treatment of MRSA-related bacteremia (39), and daptomycin is noninferior to vancomycin for right-sided endocarditis (42). Numerous reports describe failures with vancomycin, and agents superior to vancomycin are sorely needed for the treatment of MRSA endocarditis (43).

Toxin-Related Staphylococcal Infections: Necrotizing Fasciitis, Necrotizing-Hemorrhagic Pneumonia, Toxic Shock Syndrome, and Scaled Skin Syndrome

There has never been a clinical trial that specifically addressed antibiotic treatment of StaphTSS; thus, we are left to treat patients on the basis of in vitro susceptibility data. Suppression of toxin production has been demonstrated with clindamycin and linezolid, and these may offer an advantage in treating patients with toxic shock syndrome (44). It should be noted that this recommendation is based solely on in vitro toxin suppression data (45), extrapolation from experimental necrotizing infections caused by group A streptococcus (46) and *Clostridium perfringens* (47), retrospective analysis (48), and recent case reports (44). The true pathogenesis of necrotizing fasciitis and necrotizing pneumonia has not been elucidated, but is associated with CA-MRSA strains producing Panton–Valentine leukocidin. Whether that toxin singly or in combination with other toxins is responsible is being actively studied. Most would agree, however, that extracellular toxins play a major role.

As such, antibiotics that suppress these toxins could provide an added advantage in the treatment of these MRSA infections.

We have recently demonstrated that nafcillin, at subinhibitory concentrations, increases the quantities of TSST-1, PVL, and α-hemolysin in both MSSA and MRSA strains, and this was related to increased and prolonged expression of mRNA for these three toxins (45). Interestingly, clindamycin and linezolid also increased toxin gene transcription but profoundly reduced the quantities of toxins produced because of their ability to suppress protein synthesis at the ribosomal level (45).

REFERENCES

1. Everett ED, McNitt TR, Rahm AE, et al. Epidemiologic investigation of methicillin resistant *Staphylococcus aureus* in a burn unit. Military Med 1978; 143:165–167.
2. Graffunder EM, Venezia RA. Risk factors associated with nosocomial methicillin-resistant *Staphylococcus aureus* (MRSA) infection including previous use of antimicrobials. J Antimicrob Chemother 2002; 49(6):999–1005.
3. Kotilainen P, Routamaa M, Peltonen R, et al. Elimination of epidemic methicillin-resistant *Staphylococcus aureus* from a university hospital and district institutions, Finland. Emerg Infect Dis 2003; 9(2):169–175.
4. Campbell AL, Bryant KA, Stover B, et al. Epidemiology of methicillin-resistant *Staphylococcus aureus* at a children's hospital. Infect Control Hosp Epidemiol 2003; 24(6):427–430.
5. Dietrich DW, Auld DB, Mermel LA. Community-acquired methicillin-resistant *Staphylococcus aureus* in southern New England children. Pediatrics 2004; 113(4):e347–e352.
6. Purcell K, Fergie JE. Exponential increase in community-acquired methicillin-resistant *Staphylococcus aureus* infections in South Texas children. Pediatr Infect Dis J 2002; 21(10):988–989.
7. Centers for Disease Control. From the centers for disease control and prevention. Four pediatric deaths from community-acquired methicillin-resistant *Staphylococcus aureus*—Minnesota and North Dakota, 1997–1999. JAMA 1999; 282(12):1123–1125.
8. Charlebois IE, Perdreau-Remington F. Molecular evidence for clonal distinction between community and nosocomial methicillin-resistant *Staphylococcus*

aureus in 536 clinical infections. Program and Abstracts of the 40th Annual Meeting of the Infectious Disease Society of America, Chicago, October 24–27, 2002:(abstr 23)48.

9. Daum RS, Ito T, Hiramatsu K, et al. A novel methicillin-resistance cassette in community-acquired methicillin-resistant *Staphylococcus aureus* isolates of diverse genetic backgrounds. J Infect Dis 2002; 186(9):1344–1347.

10. Moran GJ, Krishnadasan A, Gorwitz RJ, et al. Methicillin-resistant *S. aureus* infections among patients in the emergency department. N Engl J Med 2006; 355(7):666–674.

11. Miller LG, Perdreau-Remington F, Rieg G, et al. Necrotizing fasciitis caused by community-associated methicillin-resistant *Staphylococcus aureus* in Los Angeles. N Engl J Med 2005; 352(14):1445–1453.

12. Francis JS, Doherty MC, Lopatin U, et al. Severe community-onset pneumonia in healthy adults caused by methicillin-resistant *Staphylococcus aureus* carrying the Panton–Valentine leukocidin genes. Clin Infect Dis 2005; 40(1):100–107.

13. Lowy FD. *Staphylococcus aureus* infections. N Engl J Med 1998; 339(8): 520–532.

14. Menzies BE, Kourteva I. *Staphylococcus aureus* alpha-toxin induces apoptosis in endothelial cells. FEMS Immunol Med Microbiol 2000; 29(1):39–45.

15. McElroy MC, Harty HR, Hosford GE, et al. Alpha-toxin damages the air-blood barrier of the lung in a rat model of *Staphylococcus aureus*-induced pneumonia. Infect Immun 1999; 67(10):5541–5544.

16. Bubeck WJ, Bae T, Otto M, et al. Poring over pores: alpha-hemolysin and Panton–Valentine leukocidin in *Staphylococcus aureus* pneumonia. Nat Med 2007; 13(12):1405–1406.

17. Bubeck WJ, Patel RJ, Schneewind O. Surface proteins and exotoxins are required for the pathogenesis of *Staphylococcus aureus* pneumonia. Infect Immun 2007; 75(2):1040–1044.

18. Bartlett AH, Foster TJ, Hayashida A, et al. Alpha-toxin facilitates the generation of CXC chemokine gradients and stimulates neutrophil homing in *Staphylococcus aureus* pneumonia. J Infect Dis 2008; 198(10):1529–1535.

19. Genestier AL, Michallet MC, Prevost G, et al. *Staphylococcus aureus* Panton–Valentine leukocidin directly targets mitochondria and induces Bax-independent apoptosis of human neutrophils. J Clin Invest 2005; 115(11): 3117–3127.

20. Dufour P, Gillet Y, Bes M, et al. Community-acquired methicillin-resistant *Staphylococcus aureus* infections in France: emergence of a single clone that produces Panton–Valentine leukocidin. Clin Infect Dis 2002; 35(7):819–824.

21. Gillet Y, Issartel B, Vanhems P, et al. Association between *Staphylococcus aureus* strains carrying gene for Panton–Valentine leukocidin and highly lethal necrotising pneumonia in young immunocompetent patients. Lancet 2002; 359(9308):753–759.

22. Lina G, Piemont Y, Godail-Gamot F, et al. Involvement of Panton–Valentine leukocidin-producing *Staphylococcus aureus* in primary skin infections and pneumonia. Clin Infect Dis 2003; 29(5):1128–1132.

23. Baggett HC, Hennessy TW, Rudolph K, et al. Community-onset methicillin-resistant *Staphylococcus aureus* associated with antibiotic use and the cytotoxin Panton–Valentine leukocidin during a furunculosis outbreak in rural Alaska. J Infect Dis 2004; 189(9):1565–1573.

24. Voyich JM, Otto M, Mathema B, et al. Is Panton–Valentine leukocidin the major virulence determinant in community-associated methicillin-resistant *Staphylococcus aureus* disease? J Infect Dis 2006; 194(12):1761–1770.

25. Labandeira-Rey M, Couzon F, Boisset S, et al. *Staphylococcus aureus* Panton–Valentine leukocidin causes necrotizing pneumonia. Science 2007; 315(5815):1130–1133.

26. Bubeck WJ, Palazzolo-Ballance AM, Otto M, et al. Panton–Valentine leukocidin is not a virulence determinant in murine models of community-associated methicillin-resistant *Staphylococcus aureus* disease. J Infect Dis 2008; 198(8):1166–1170.

27. Pannaraj PS, Hulten KG, Gonzalez BE, et al. Infective pyomyositis and myositis in children in the era of community-acquired, methicillin-resistant *Staphylococcus aureus* infection. Clin Infect Dis 2006; 43(8):953–960.

28. Naimi TS, LeDell KH, Como-Sabetti K, et al. Comparison of community- and health care-associated methicillin-resistant *Staphylococcus aureus* infection. JAMA 2003; 290(22):2976–2984.

29. Hamilton SM, Bryant AE, Carroll KC, et al. In vitro production of Panton–Valentine leukocidin (PVL) among strains of methicillin-resistant *Staphylococcus aureus* causing diverse infections. Clin Infect Dis 2007; 45(12): 1550–1558.

30. Furukawa Y, Segawa Y, Masuda K, et al. [Clinical experience of 3 cases of toxic shock syndrome caused by methicillin cephem-resistant *Staphylococcus aureus* (MRSA)]. Kansenshogaku Zasshi 1986; 60(10):1147–1153.

31. Schmitz FJ, MacKenzie CR, Geisel R, et al. Enterotoxin and toxic shock syndrome toxin-1 production of methicillin resistant and methicillin sensitive *Staphylococcus aureus* strains. Eur J Epidemiol 1997; 13(6):699–708.

32. Meyer RD, Monday SR, Bohach GA, et al. Prolonged course of toxic shock syndrome associated with methicillin-resistant *Staphylococcus aureus* enterotoxins G and I. Int J Infect Dis 2001; 5(3):163–166.

33. Kikuchi K, Takahashi N, Piao C, et al. Molecular epidemiology of methicillin-resistant *Staphylococcus aureus* strains causing neonatal toxic shock syndrome-like exanthematous disease in neonatal and perinatal wards. J Clin Microbiol 2003; 41(7):3001–3006.

34. van der Mee-Marquet N, Epinette C, Loyau J, et al. *Staphylococcus aureus* strains isolated from bloodstream infections changed significantly in 2006. J Clin Microbiol 2007; 45(3):851–857.

35. Jamart S, Denis O, Deplano A, et al. Methicillin-resistant *Staphylococcus aureus* toxic shock syndrome. Emerg Infect Dis 2005; 11(4):636–637.

36. Fujiwara Y, Endo S. A case of toxic shock syndrome secondary to mastitis caused by methicillin-resistant *Staphylococcus aureus*. Kansenshogaku Zasshi 2001; 75(10):898–903.

37. Amano T, Imao T, Fukuda M, et al. Toxic shock syndrome due to methicillin resistant *Staphylococcus aureus* (MRSA) after total prostatectomy. Nippon Hinyokika Gakkai Zasshi 2002; 93(1):44–47.

38. Nakano M, Miyazawa H, Kawano Y, et al. An outbreak of neonatal toxic shock syndrome-like exanthematous disease (NTED) caused by methicillin-resistant *Staphylococcus aureus* (MRSA) in a neonatal intensive care unit. Microbiol Immunol 2002; 46(4):277–284.

39. Stevens DL, Herr D, Lampiris H, et al. Linezolid versus vancomycin for the treatment of methicillin-resistant *Staphylococcus aureus* infections. Clin Infect Dis 2002; 34:1481–1490.

40. Plouffe JF. Emerging therapies for serious gram-positive bacterial infections: a focus on linezolid. Clin Infect Dis 2000; 31(suppl 4):S144–S149.

41. Conte J, Golden JA, Kipps J, et al. Intrapulmonary pharmacokinetics of linezolid. Antimicrob Agents Chemother 2002; 46(5):1475–1480.

42. Fowler VG Jr., Boucher HW, Corey GR, et al. Daptomycin versus standard therapy for bacteremia and endocarditis caused by *Staphylococcus aureus*. N Engl J Med 2006; 355(7):653–665.

43. Gonzalez C, Rubio M, Romero-Vivas J, et al. Bacteremic pneumonia due to *Staphylococcus aureus*: a comparison of disease caused by methicillin-resistant and methicillin-susceptible organisms. Clin Infect Dis 1999; 29(5): 1171–1177.

44. Stevens DL, Wallace RJ, Hamilton SM, et al. Successful treatment of staphylococcal toxic shock syndrome with linezolid: a case report and in vitro

evaluation of the production of toxic shock syndrome toxin type 1 in the presence of antibiotics. Clin Infect Dis 2006; 42(5):729–730.

45. Stevens DL, Ma Y, Salmi DB, et al. Impact of antibiotics on expression of virulence-associated exotoxin genes in methicillin-sensitive and methicillin-resistant *Staphylococcus aureus*. J Infect Dis 2007; 195(2):202–211.

46. Stevens DL, Bryant-Gibbons AE, Bergstrom R, et al. The Eagle effect revisited: efficacy of clindamycin, erythromycin, and penicillin in the treatment of streptococcal myositis. J Infect Dis 1988; 158:23–28.

47. Stevens DL, Maier KA, Mitten JE. Effect of antibiotics on toxin production and viability of *Clostridium perfringens*. Antimicrob Agents Chemother 1987; 31:213–218.

48. Zimbelman J, Palmer A, Todd J. Improved outcome of clindamycin compared with beta-lactam antibiotic treatment for invasive *Streptococcus pyogenes* infection. Pediatr Infect Dis J 1999; 18(12):1096–1100.

Community-Associated MRSA as a Pathogen

4

Karen J. Brasel and John A. Weigelt
Department of Surgery, Medical College of Wisconsin, Milwaukee, Wisconsin, U.S.A.

INTRODUCTION

Community-associated methicillin-resistant *Staphylococcus aureus* (CA-MRSA) was initially defined as an infection with methicillin-resistant *S. aureus* (MRSA) in an outpatient or in a patient that manifested infection within 48 hours of hospital admission (1). It was soon recognized that CA-MRSA has unique characteristics not related to time of onset or hospitalization that differentiate it from health care–associated MRSA (HA-MRSA). These include epidemiology, presentation, treatment, and genetic profile.

The CDC defined a new classification system for MRSA infections in 2007 (2). MRSA infections were divided into health care–associated and community-associated infections based on epidemiologic investigations. Table 1 lists the characteristics of each category.

This classification is helpful for epidemiologic studies, but there are other important clinical differences between the two organisms. CA-MRSA infections primarily affect skin and skin structures. HA-MRSA infections can involve skin structures but are commonly seen in the respiratory tract, urinary tract, and bloodstream. Treatment options are also different since CA-MRSA strains are not multidrug resistant like HA-MRSA. Most CA-MRSA strains are susceptible to non-β-lactam antibiotics.

Additionally, there are genetic differences between CA-MRSA and HA-MRSA. Most CA-MRSA in the United States are typed as USA300 while USA100 is the most frequent HA-MRSA.

TABLE 1 Epidemiologic Classification of MRSA Infections

Classification	Definition
Health care associated	
Community onset	Must have at least one of the following health care risk factors: 1. An invasive device in place at time of admission 2. History of MRSA infection or colonization 3. History of surgery, dialysis, hospitalization, or residence in long-term care facility, in the previous 12 mo
Hospital onset	Positive culture after 48 hr of hospitalization with or without community onset risk factors
Community associated	Cases with no documented risk factors

Abbreviation: MRSA, methicillin-resistant *Staphylococcus aureus*.

EPIDEMIOLOGY

The original outbreak of CA-MRSA was described in a U.S. population of intravenous drug users, and CA-MRSA infections were initially restricted to specific patient populations (3). Patients in closed populations predominated, including Native Americans, men who have sex with men, prison inmates, children in daycare centers, military recruits, and competitive athletes in team sports (3–6). However, the prevalence of CA-MRSA has increased to the point that the majority of infections occur in patients without these risk factors. CA-MRSA has become an international problem, with infection and colonization spreading worldwide (4,6–10).

    In the United States, the prevalence of MRSA in the general population was estimated from the 2001–2002 NHANES (National

Health and Nutrition Examination Survey) data. The overall colonization rate of noninstitutionalized persons with methicillin-sensitive *S. aureus* is 31.6% and 0.84% with MRSA. Incidence rates of invasive CA-MRSA infection range from 1.6/100,000 to 29.7/100,000 population (2).

Current estimates of CA-MRSA prevalence vary from 5% to 76% (11,12). These estimates vary by patient population and clinical situation. Screening programs place the colonization rate of patients entering the hospital at 5% (13). Reports from emergency departments identify CA-MRSA as the etiologic agent in 76% of patients with skin and skin structure infections (14). On the basis of retrospective studies, the proportion of MRSA infections attributable to CA-MRSA is approximately 30%. In prospective series the incidence is somewhat higher, approximately 38% (1). In a rigorous MRSA surveillance program, CA-MRSA is responsible for 5% to 30% of invasive MRSA infections; the incidence varies significantly depending on location (2). There is some evidence that CA-MRSA is responsible for an increasing proportion of invasive MRSA infections (15), and in some areas the prevalence of the disease in the community is now greater than it is in the hospital (16).

Risk factors associated with HA-MRSA infection guided recommendations for empiric MRSA treatment in high-risk hospitalized patients. Unfortunately, the majority of these risk factors are not present in patients with CA-MRSA. Perhaps of greater concern, it is difficult to distinguish patients with CA-MRSA infection from those with MSSA infection on the basis of epidemiologic characteristics (17). This suggests that at a minimum, knowledge of local prevalence rates and sites of infection should guide treatment. However, even in an area with low CA-MRSA prevalence (10%), patients lacking the three strongest risk factors still have a 7% posttest probability of CA-MRSA infection (17). These data have important implications from an infection control standpoint as well as in guiding treatment recommendations.

As the prevalence of CA-MRSA has increased, isolation of this organism from SSIs (surgical site infections) has also increased. Up to 25%

of SSIs are caused by CA-MRSA (18,19). Surgical prophylaxis targeting *S. aureus* routinely uses a first-generation cephalosporin. The increasing CA-MRSA rates for SSIs has raised the question of proper screening and altering drug choices, although no firm recommendations are being promulgated at this time.

Bacterial Characteristics

The hallmark of both CA-MRSA and HA-MRSA is methicillin and β-lactam resistance, mediated by the altered penicillin-binding protein 2a. The gene responsible for methicillin resistance, *mecA*, is located on a mobile chromosomal element called the staphylococcal cassette chromosome (SCCmec). There are five known types of the staphylococcal cassette chromosome (SCC). Types I, II, and III, found in HA-MRSA, are relatively large and carry resistance to many different antibiotics. In contrast, CA-MRSA carries predominantly type IV (20,21). Type IV SCC was described in 2002 and is a much smaller SCC that lacks many of the other resistance genes common in IIA-MRSA. SCCmec type V has recently been found in some strains of CA-MRSA from Australia (22).

SCCmec type IV was identified from isolates of *S. epidermidis* in the 1970s (23). Although CA-MRSA was described in an isolated outbreak in the late 1970s, widespread findings of CA-MRSA did not occur until 1989, suggesting that methicillin resistance may have originated in coagulase-negative bacteria. The small size of SCCmec type IV, in contrast to types II and III, likely contributes to the diversity of CA-MRSA strains as horizontal transfer of the small element is easily accomplished.

The Panton–Valentine leukocidin (PVL) gene was initially identified as the most clinically significant virulence factors in CA-MRSA. The PVL gene, initially described in 1894 and further characterized by Panton and Valentine in 1932, encodes a pore-forming cytotoxin that acts preferentially against leukocytes and erythrocytes (24). It is commonly found in CA-MRSA infections and only rarely in HA-MRSA. In an epidemiologic study from Minnesota, it was present in 77% of all CA-MRSA and in only 4% of HA-MRSA (25). Although commonly found in CA-MRSA, the PVL gene is not genetically linked to SCCmec type IV. The PVL gene is found in methicillin-sensitive *S. aureus* and clearly predates the development of methicillin resistance, suggesting that CA-MRSA arose via transfer of SCCmec type IV into methicillin-sensitive strains of *S. aureus* with the PVL gene (5).

The role of PVL toxin in the pathogenesis of CA-MRSA skin and soft-tissue infections (SSTIs) is unclear. Similar skin infections are reported in PVL-negative strains (26). Numerous other virulence genes are identified (27). A group of peptides have also been identified that are secreted by CA-MRSA (28). They can recruit, activate and lyse human neutrophils which are the main defense against *S. aureus* infection. These appear to be another component in promoting CA-MRSA virulence.

PVL toxin is suggested as having a greater role in the pathogenesis of pneumonia. PVL-positive MRSA pneumonia is reported following influenza-like illness in immunocompetent patients. PVL positivity was associated with a 94% mortality rate at 48 hours compared to a 63% mortality rate when the MRSA was PVL negative (29,30).

PRESENTATION

The majority of infections caused by CA-MRSA are SSTIs, accounting for approximately 75% of infections in adults and up to 90% of pediatric infections (25,31,32). In one urban hospital, CA-MRSA SSTIs increased from 24 cases/100,000 people in 2000 to 164.2 cases/100,000 people in a five-year period (33). Clinical presentation of these infections may vary from minor cellulitis to necrotizing soft-tissue infections. Abscesses are the most common manifestation. Lesions may be single or multiple, and satellite lesions are often present. The cytotoxicity conferred by exotoxin genes can result in an intense inflammatory cascade and extensive tissue necrosis. The resulting skin lesion can mimic a brown

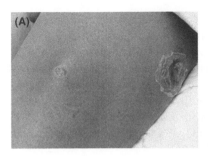
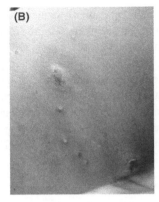

FIGURE 1 (**A**, **B**) Community-acquired MRSA infection of the thigh showing multiple lesions. A typical lesion has central necroses, surrounding induration, which is encircled by cellulitis.

recluse spider bite with central necrosis, surrounding induration and erythema (Fig. 1). However, even within areas where the brown recluse spider is endemic, lesions are much more likely because of CA-MRSA than spider bites (34).

Pneumonia is the second most common clinical manifestation of CA-MRSA. Many of these pneumonias are necrotizing because of the presence of PVL gene. This results in mucosal ulcerations as well as hemorrhagic necrosis of the interalveolar septa. The role of PVL in the pathogenesis of CA-MRSA pneumonia is much clearer than its role in SSTIs (35). PVL-positive strains of *S. aureus* bind preferentially to damaged respiratory epithelium, explaining the association with prior influenza-like illnesses (36,37). In the 2003–2004 influenza season, 19 cases of CA-MRSA pneumonia were reported in the United States in patients with documented or suspected influenza preceding the MRSA infection. Fourteen of 15 isolates tested expressed the PVL toxin (37).

The potentially virulent nature of CA-MRSA infections was realized in the late 1990s, with the report of four fatalities in pediatric patients without previous risk factors (38). One patient suffered from a septic right hip, another meningitis, and two patients had pneumonia. Three patients were bacteremic at the time of their death. A variety of other infections, including osteomyelitis and meningitis, have now been reported to be because of CA-MRSA. In patients with pneumonia, presence of the PVL gene results in a much higher mortality, 37% compared to 6% for patients with PVL-negative pneumonia (7).

TREATMENT

Unlike HA-MRSA where the large SCCmec types I to III encode multiple resistance genes, SCCmec types IV and V encode relatively few. The most common strain of CA-MRSA causing skin infection in the United States is USA300-0114. USA300-0114 is resistant to four antimicrobial agents other than methicillin and penicillin. The most common pattern included resistance to erythromycin, found in over 90%. A separate plasmid encodes for tetracycline resistance, which occurred in 23% of isolates. Inducible resistance to levofloxacin was present in 20%. Clindamycin resistance, which can be either inducible or constitutive, is encoded by another plasmid and was present in 13%. The combination of resistance to all four additional antimicrobial agents was not described (39). Resistance patterns differ notably by geographic region, with clindamycin resistance more prevalent in the southern United States (39,40).

A variety of oral agents are available to treat mild-to-moderate infections with CA-MRSA on the basis of resistance patterns for the bacteria. Trimethoprim-sulfamethoxazole and doxycycline are both acceptable, as the resistance rates to both of these agents are low. The efficacy of expanded-spectrum tetracyclines has been confirmed in a retrospective series (41). A prospective trial of doxycycline and trimethoprim-sulfamethoxazole showed statistical equivalency, although all treatment failures occurred in the trimethoprim group (42). Neither agent has activity against streptococci—potentially problematic in treating cellulitis or other infections where the causative gram-positive agent may not be known. Clindamycin has broader activity against gram-positive infections, but must be used with some caution because of the potential for inducible resistance. Inducible resistance is not found in strains that are susceptible to erythromycin; however, the majority of strains responsible for soft-tissue infections are erythromycin resistant. Inducible clindamycin resistance can be detected by using the double-disk diffusion test (D-test). This test was recommended as the standard by the Clinical and Laboratory Standards Institute (CLSI, formerly NCCLS) in 2004 and is now a routine in many laboratories, but can delay results of susceptibility testing by 24 to 48 hours (40).

Severe or invasive infections due to CA-MRSA require hospitalization and intravenous antibiotics. Intravenous forms of the aforementioned antimicrobials are effective for these infections, although they should be used only if HA-MRSA is not a concern. If HA-MRSA is a possibility, vancomycin, daptomycin, linezolid, tigecycline, or quinupristin-dalfopristin (not Food and Drug Administration–approved for MRSA) should be used until results of sensitivity testing are available. Whether agents that shut down toxin production, such as clindamycin, tetracycline, and linezolid, are specifically more effective in toxin-producing strains of CA-MRSA infection is unknown. Linezolid is more effective than vancomycin in treating both pneumonia and complicated skin and soft-tissue infections because of the combination of CA-MRSA and HA-MRSA (41). It is unclear whether this will remain true for pneumonia and soft-tissue infections due solely to CA-MRSA.

Resistance patterns, in addition to varying by geographic region, also vary by age. In a group of patients treated at the University of Chicago, erythromycin, clindamycin, ciprofloxacin, gentamicin, and tetracycline resistance was much more common in adult patients than pediatric patients. Particularly striking was the difference in resistance to clindamycin: 52% in adults compared to 7% in pediatric patients (42). This has led to the use of clindamycin as a first-line agent in many CA-MRSA infections in the pediatric population.

One of the hallmarks of CA-MRSA infections has been inadequate initial antibiotic therapy, usually with a β-lactam agent (25). This occurs because the majority of patients with CA-MRSA infections do not have risk factors, triggering the clinician's concern for possible MRSA infection. Knowledge of endemic rates of CA-MRSA, careful assessment of potential risk factors, and recognition of lesions typical of CA-MRSA are all necessary to ensure adequacy of initial treatment. In our experience, CA-MRSA should be suspected in any patient with a skin lesion that has central necrosis, surrounding erythema and a large amount of induration. Satellite lesions should increase suspicion for a CA-MRSA infection. Despite the increased recognition of CA-MRSA as an important pathogen and use of appropriate empiric antibiotics (43), in some places the majority of patients with CA-MRSA SSTIs are still treated with inadequate initial antibiotics (44).

Surgical treatment has been the standard treatment for soft-tissue abscesses, including those because of CA-MRSA and HA-MRSA. Incision and drainage is recommended, with concomitant antibiotic therapy indicated for surrounding cellulitis or systemic illness. Healthy patients with small abscesses and no surrounding cellulitis may be treated with incision and drainage alone (35).

Perhaps because of the presence of an exotoxin gene in many of these infections, small abscesses contain a minimal amount of drainable material; the majority of the infection or "abscess" is an intense inflammatory reaction. Rather than multiple incisions that yield minimal results in these very small abscesses, the authors have had good success in treating adult patients with oral antibiotics and close follow-up. The typical course is a lesion that dries up over the course of five to seven days. A patient is usually treated for five days and reevaluated. Longer courses are rarely needed despite the 10- to 12-day duration reported in the largest MRSA complicated skin and skin structure study (41). Treatment failures after five to seven days may need surgical drainage. Ultrasound is helpful in identifying lesions that can benefit from drainage. Ultrasound can be used initially or in those patients that do not resolve their lesion after five to seven days. Often no drainable fluid is present and longer courses of antibiotics are needed. Treatment failures may also be secondary to drug resistance. If no improvement occurs after five days, then use of an HA-MRSA drug is the authors' approach. Oral therapy is commonly continued with linezolid in patients who fail initial therapy with either doxycycline or clindamycin. Hospitalization is rarely indicated if the correct diagnosis is made and the patient has no systemic signs of toxicity.

PREVENTION

Standard infection control principles are the best method to prevent outbreaks because of CA-MRSA. These include hand washing, daily showers, use of antibacterial soap, covering any draining lesions, isolation of infected patients needing hospitalization, and avoidance of sharing personal items. Isolation may require withholding athletes with draining wounds from competition and not allowing health care workers with open wounds to return to work until they have healed (6). Contact isolation procedures should be used for hospitalized patients.

Immunization has been attempted in high-risk dialysis patients (45). Partial immunity was achieved, but it did not last. No vaccine is approved for clinical use at this time. Decolonization has been attempted both for outbreak control and to prevent recurrence. Various strategies, including systemic antibiotics, chlorhexidine body washes, and mupiricin nasal ointment, have been tried with limited effectiveness. Although there are insufficient data to recommend any one strategy over another, decolonization is probably worthwhile in high-risk patient populations and with recurrent disease in an individual or in families (6,46).

CONCLUSIONS

It is clear that understanding the role CA-MRSA plays in staphylococcal disease is important to the clinician. CA-MRSA is clearly different from HA-MRSA. Although the population prevalence of asymptomatic colonization in the United States is relatively low, it has increased over time and will likely continue to increase. The proportion of staphylococcal infections because of CA-MRSA has reached the point where empiric coverage against this pathogen should be considered in many cases. Recognition of typical skin lesions, pneumonia associated with influenza-like illnesses, and knowledge of local prevalence rates will help institute appropriate therapy early.

REFERENCES

1. Salgado CD, Farr BM, Calfee DP. Community-acquired methicillin-resistant *Staphylococcus aureus*: a meta-analysis of prevalence and risk factors. Clin Infect Dis 2003; 36:131–139.
2. Klevens RM, Morrison MA, et al. Invasive methicillin-resistant *Staphylococcus aureus* infections in the United States. JAMA 2007; 298:1763–1771.
3. Saravolatz LD, Markowitz N, Arking L, et al. Epidemiologic observations during a community-acquired outbreak. Ann Intern Med 1982; 96:11–16.
4. Gosbell IB. Epidemiology, clinical features and management of infections due to community methicillin-resistant *Staphylococcus aureus* (cMRSA). Int Med J 2005; 35:S120–S135.
5. Nolte O, Haag H, Zimmerman A, et al. *Staphylococcus aureus* positive for Panton–Valentine leukocidin genes but susceptible to methicillin in patients with furuncles. Eur J Clin Microbiol Infect Dis 2005; 24:477–479.
6. Kowalski TJ, Berbari EF, Osmon DR. Epidemiology, treatment, and prevention of community-acquired methicillin-resistant *Staphylococcus aureus* infections. Mayo Clin Proc 2005; 80:1201–1208.
7. Kollef MH, Micek ST. Methicillin-resistant *Staphylococcus aureus*: a new community-acquired pathogen? Curr Opinion Infect Dis 2006; 19:161–168.
8. von Specht M, Gardella N, Tagliaferri P, et al. Methicillin-resistant *Staphylococcus aureus* in community-acquired meningitis. Eur J Clin Microbiol Infect Dis 2006; 25:267–269.

9. Naas T, Fortineau N, Spicq C, et al. Three-year survey of community-acquired methicillin-resistant *Staphylococcus aureus* producing Panton–Valentine leukocidin in a French university hospital. J Hosp Infect 2006; 61:321–329.

10. Kluytmans-VendenBergh MFQ, Kluytmans JAJW. Community-acquired methicillin-resistant *Staphylococcus aureus*: current perspectives. Clin Micro Infect 2006; 12:9–15.

11. Fridkin SK, Hageman JC, Morrison M, et al. Methicillin-resistant *Staphylococcus aureus* disease in three communities. N Engl J Med 2005; 352: 1436–1444.

12. Folden DV, Machayya JA, Sahmoun AE, et al. Estimating the proportion of community-associated methicillin-resistant *Staphylococcus aureus*: two definitions used in the USA yield dramatically different estimates. J Hosp Infect 2005; 60:329–332.

13. Robicsek A, Beaumont JL, Paule SM, et al. Universal surveillance for methicillin-resistant *Staphylococcus aureus* in 3 affiliated hospitals. Ann Intern Med 2008; 148:409–418.

14. Moran GJ, Krishnadasan A, Gorwitz RJ, et al. Methicillin-resistant *S. aureus* infections among patients in the emergency department. N Engl J Med 2006; 355:666–674.

15. Popovich KJ, Weinstein RA, Hota B. Are community-associated methicillin-resistant *Staphylococcus aureus* (MRSA) strains replacing traditional nosocomial MRSA strains? Clin Infect Dis 2008; 46:787–794.

16. Liu C, Graber CJ, Karr M, et al. A population-based study of the incidence molecular epidemiology of methicillin-resistant *Staphylococcus aureus* disease in San Francisco, 2004–2005. Clin Infect Dis 2008; 46:1637–1646.

17. Miller LG, Perdreau-Remington F, Bayer AS, et al. Clinical and epidemiology characteristics cannot distinguish community-associated methicillin-resistant *Staphylococcus aureus* infection from methicillin-susceptible *S. aureus* infection: a prospective investigation. Clin Infect Dis 2007; 44:471–482.

18. Awad SS, Elhabash SI, Lee L, et al. Increasing incidence of methicillin-resistant *Staphylococcus aureus* skin and soft-tissue infections: reconsideration of empiric antimicrobial therapy. Am J Surg 2007; 194:606–610.

19. Lipsky BA, Weigelt JA, Gupta V, et al. Skin, soft tissue, bone, and joint infections in hospitalized patients: epidemiology and microbiological, clinical, and economic outcomes. Infect Control Hosp Epidemiol 2007; 28:1290–1298.

20. Tenover FC, McDougal LK, Goering RV. Characterization of a strain of community-associated methicillin-resistant *Staphylococcus aureus* widely disseminated in the United States. J Clin Micro 2006; 44:108–118.

21. Ma XX, Ito T, Tiensasitorn C, et al. Novel type of staphylococcal cassette chromosome mec identified in community-acquired methicillin-resistant *Staphylococcus aureus* strains. Antimicrob Agents Chemother 2002; 46:1147–1152.
22. O'Brien FG, Coombs GW, Pearson JC, et al. Type V staphylococcal cassette chromosome mec in community staphylococci from Australia. Antimicrob Agents Chemother 2005; 49:5129–5132.
23. Wisplinghoff H, Rosato AE, Enright MC, et al. Related clones containing SCCmec type IV predominate among clinically significant *Staphylococcus epidermidis* isolates. Antimicrob Agents Chemother 2003; 47:3574–3579.
24. Panton PN, Valentine FCO. Staphylococcal toxin. Lancet 1932; 1:506–508.
25. Naimi TS, LeDell KN, Como-Sabetti K, et al. Comparison of community-and health care-associated methicillin-resistant *Staphylococcus aureus* infection. J Am Med Assoc 2003; 290:2976–2984.
26. Voyich JM, Otto M, Mathema B, et al. Is Panton–Valentine leukocidin the major virulence determinant in community-associated methicillin-resistant *Staphylococcus aureus* disease? J Infect Dis 2006; 194:1761–170.
27. An Diep B, Carleton HA, Chang RF, et al. Roles of 34 virulence genes in the evolution of hospital- and community-associated strains of methicillin-resistant *Staphylococcus aureus*. J Iinfect Dis 2006; 193:1495–1503.
28. Wang R, Braughton KR, Kretschmer D, et al. Identification of novel cytolytic peptides as key virulence determinants for community-associated MRSA. Nat Med 2007; 13:1510–1514.
29. Gillet Y, Issartel B, Vanhems P, et al. Association between *Staphylococcus aureus* strains carrying gene for Panton–Valentine leukocidin and highly lethal necrotizing pneumonia in young immunocompetent patients. Lancet 2002; 359:753–759.
30. Labandeira-Rey M, Couzon F, Boisset S, et al. *Staphylococcus aureus* Panton–Valentine leukocidin causes necrotizing pneumonia. Science 2007; 315:1130–1133.
31. Kaplan SL. Implications of methicillin-resistant *Staphylococcus aureus* as a community-acquired pathogen in pediatric patients. Infect Dis Clin N Am 2005; 19:747–757.
32. Jungk J, Como-Sabetti K, Stinchfield P, et al. Epidemiology of methicillin-resistant *Staphylococcus aureus* at a pediatric healthcare system, 1991–2003. Ped Infect Dis J 2007; 26:339–344.
33. Hota B, Ellenbogen C, Hayden MK, et al. Community-associated methicillin-resistant *Staphylococcus aureus* skin and soft tissue infections at a public hospital. Arch Intern Med 2007; 167:1026–1033.

34. Swanson DL, Vetter RS. Bites of brown recluse spiders and suspected necrotic arachnidism. N Engl J Med 2005; 352:700–707.
35. Stryjewski ME, Chambers HF. Skin and soft-tissue infections caused by community-acquired methicillin-resistant *Staphylococcus aureus*. Clin Infect Dis 2008; 46:S368–S377.
36. Francis JS, Doherty MC, Lopatin U, et al. Severe community-onset pneumonia in healthy adults caused by methicillin-resistant *Staphylococcus aureus* carrying the Panton–Valentine leukocidin genes. Clin Infect Dis 2005; 40:100–107.
37. Hageman JC, Uyeki TM, Francis JS, et al. Severe community-acquired pneumonia due to *Staphylococcus aureus*, 2003–2004 influenza season. Emerg Infect Dis 2006; 12:894–899.
38. MMWR 1999; 48:707–710.
39. King MD, Humphrey BJ, Wang YF, et al. Emergence of community-acquired methicillin-resistant *Staphylococcus aureus* USA300 clone as the predominant cause of skin and soft-tissue infections. Ann Intern Med 2006; 144:309–317.
40. Lewis JS, Jorgensen JH. Inducible clindamycin resistance in staphylococci: should clinicians and microbiologists be concerned? Clin Infect Dis 2005; 40:280–285.
41. Weigelt JA, Itani K, Stevens D, et al. Linezolid versus vancomycin in treatment of complicated skin and soft tissue infections. Antimicrob Agents Chemother 2005; 49:2260–2266.
42. David MZ, Crawford SE, Boyle-Vavra S, et al. Contrasting pediatric and adult methicillin-resistant *Staphylococcus aureus* isolates. Emerg Infect Dis 2006; 12:631–637.
43. Pallin DJ, Egan DJ, Pelletier AJ, et al. Increased US Emergency Department visits for skin and soft tissue infections, and changes in antibiotic choices, during the emergence of community-associated methicillin-resistant *Staphylococcus aureus*. Ann Emerg Med 2008; 51:291–298.
44. Ruhe JJ, Menon A. Tetracyclines as an oral treatment option for patients with community-onset skin and soft tissue infections caused by methicillin-resistant *Staphylococcus aureus*. Antimicrob Agents Chemo 2007; 51:3298–3303.
45. Shinefield H, Black S, Fattom A, et al. Use of a *Staphylococcus aureus* conjugate vaccine in patients receiving hemodialysis. N Engl J Med 2002; 346:491–496.
46. Khoury J, Jones M, Grim A, et al. Eradication of methicillin-resistant *Staphylococcus aureus* from a neonatal intensive care unit by active surveillance and aggressive infection control measures. Infect Control Hosp Epidemiol 2005; 26:616–621.

MRSA and Complicated Skin and Soft Tissue Infections

5

Kamal M. F. Itani
Boston Veterans Affairs Health Care System, Boston University, Boston, Massachusetts, U.S.A.

DEFINITION

Infections involving skin and soft tissue are referred to by two synonymous terms: skin and skin structure infections and skin and soft tissue infections (SSTIs), complicated or uncomplicated (1). Uncomplicated SSTIs include superficial infections, such as cellulitis, simple abscesses, impetigo, and furuncles. In most instances, these infections can be treated by surgical incision alone or in the case of cellulitis with antibiotics alone.

The complicated SSTI (cSSTI) category includes infections either involving deeper soft tissue or requiring significant surgical intervention, such as infected ulcers, burns, and major abscesses, or a significant underlying disease state and comorbidities that complicate the response to treatment. Superficial infections or abscesses in an anatomical site, such as the rectal area, where the risk of anaerobic or gram-negative pathogen involvement is higher, should be considered complicated infections (1). SSTIs in critical anatomical locations such as the face and periorbital areas as well as the neck, hands, and feet should also be considered complicated.

For uncomplicated SSTIs, the two most common pathogens are *Streptococcus pyogenes* and *Staphylococcus aureus* with community-acquired MRSA (CA-MRSA) becoming a leading cause of these infections (2). Other isolated organisms are not uniformly considered pathogens in this condition, but rather seen as colonizers or contaminants. For cSSTI, the possible pathogens are numerous and dependent on the clinical situation, the location of the lesion/infection, and past medical history of the patient. In addition, it is sometimes difficult to separate a colonizer from a pathogen, since the same organism can be either one, depending on the clinical setting (1).

There is a continuum from contamination to colonization and finally infection. Contamination has no signs of local or systemic response. As the wound becomes progressively colonized with rising bacterial counts, subtle local signs occur, signaling a change in the equilibrium or an increasing bioburden contributing to abnormal wound homeostasis, and possible delayed healing. Infection occurs when the bacteria have invaded the tissue, are multiplying, and cause a systemic host reaction and impaired healing. While infection in acute wounds may be easy to identify, the chronic colonized wound often presents a challenge when trying to identify signs and symptoms of infection.

Staphylococcal cSSTI can be caused by methicillin-sensitive *S. aureus* (MSSA) or methicillin-resistant *S. aureus* (MRSA) bacteria. A recent increase in prevalence of MRSA cSSTI has caused a reevaluation of treatment principles.

COMMUNITY-ACQUIRED AND HEALTH CARE–RELATED MRSA IN SKIN AND SOFT TISSUE INFECTIONS

Until recently, drug-resistant strains of *S. aureus* were considered to be acquired almost exclusively in hospital settings, but reports of MRSA acquired in the community are increasing, and are most often associated with SSTI. In the SENTRY antimicrobial surveillance program, *S. aureus* was found to be the predominant pathogen in nosocomial SSTI, accounting for 51.6% of the isolates in North America. Among the *S. aureus* isolates, 47% were methicillin resistant (3). These data collected in 2004 show a significant increase in the MRSA rate of 30% in 2000 (4). The overall MRSA rate in North America is highest (35.9%), compared to Latin America (29.4%) and Europe (22.8%) (3).

In a prospective cohort study of MRSA cases conducted in Minnesota in the year 2000, 12% of the strains were CA-MRSA, accounting for 75% of all SSTI in that population (5). Although CA-MRSA is usually resistant to the β-lactam group of antibiotics, it is usually susceptible in vitro to fluoroquinolones, trimethoprim/sulfamethoxazole, clindamycin, and chloramphenicol. This is in contradistinction to health care–acquired MRSA (HA-MRSA), which is usually resistant to fluoroquinolones, clindamycin, and chloramphenicol, and is less sensitive to trimethoprim/sulfamethoxazole. Clusters of CA-MRSA cSSTI have been documented among athletes participating in contact sports, military recruits, Pacific Islanders, Alaskan natives, Native Americans, men who have sex with men, IV drug users, and prisoners (6). Correctional inmates with HIV infections are twice as likely to develop MRSA infections compared with HIV-negative inmates (6). Factors associated with the spread of CA-MRSA skin infections in otherwise healthy people include close skin-to-skin contact, openings in the skin such as cuts or abrasions, contaminated items and surfaces, crowded living conditions, and poor hygiene. In a case-controlled study, persons with CA-MRSA SSTI had received significantly more courses of antibiotics in the year before the outbreak (a median of 4 vs. 2 courses, $p = 0.01$) (7).

Risk factors for HA-MRSA infection include a current or recent hospitalization, residing in a long-term care facility, previous infection with MRSA, chronic wounds, and patients with invasive devices, such as dialysis, Foley catheters, feeding tubes, and intravenous catheters.

SIGNS AND SYMPTOMS

Infections with *S. aureus*, including MRSA, generally start as small, red bumps that resemble pimples. They can become deep, painful abscesses that require surgical drainage. Most of the time, the bacteria remain confined to the skin, but they can cause potentially life-threatening infections in bones, joints, surgical wounds, the bloodstream, heart valves, and lungs. Unlike HA-MRSA, CA-MRSA is more likely to produce the Panton-Valentine leukocidin toxin that destroys white blood cells and living tissue. The toxin can cause severe, often fatal skin infections (necrotizing fasciitis) and pneumonia.

Necrotizing Skin and Soft Tissue Infection

Necrotizing fasciitis is a rapidly progressive, life-threatening infection involving the skin, soft tissue, and deep fascia. These infections are typically caused by a group A *Streptococcus*, *Clostridium perfringens*, or a mixture of aerobic and anaerobic organisms, typically including group A *Streptococcus*, the enterobacteriaceae, and anaerobes. In the past, *S. aureus* has been a very uncommon cause of necrotizing fasciitis, but CA-MRSA is an emerging cause of necrotizing fasciitis (8). In a recent report of 14 patients with MRSA necrotizing fasciitis, necrotizing myositis, or both, the median age was 46 years and 71% were men. Coexisting or risk factors included current or past infection, drug use (43%), previous MRSA infection, diabetes, and chronic hepatitis C (21% each). Wound cultures were monomicrobial for MRSA in 86% of cases. All MRSA isolates were susceptible in vitro to clindamycin, trimethoprim/sulfamethoxazole, and rifampin. All recovered isolates were mec type IV and carried the Panton-Valentine leukocidin gene. The author suggests that in areas where CA-MRSA infections are endemic, empirical therapy for MRSA infection should not be withheld from patients with suspected necrotizing fasciitis on the basis of the absence of clinical risk factors. This is a distinct change in the approach to the patient with a necrotizing skin and soft tissue infection, as therapy against CA-MRSA is not currently recommended for these patients (8).

Surgical Site Infection

Infections of surgical wounds are the most common adverse events affecting hospitalized patients who have undergone surgery. Recent data from the Centers for Disease Control show a 2.6% incidence of surgical site infections (SSIs), although this incidence is believed to be higher because of inadequate postdischarge surveillance (9). The frequency of SSI is related to the category of operation, with clean and low-risk operations having the lowest rate of infection and contamination and high-risk operations having greater infection rates. Scoring systems have been developed to predict the risk of SSI, the most popular of which is the one developed by the National Nosocomial Infection Surveillance (NNIS) (10). Data for the NNIS system were derived from 44 participating hospitals and conducted by the CDC. Traditional wound class of contaminated or dirty/infected wounds was maintained as one of the factors used to predict risk for wound infection. The American Society of Anesthesiologists (ASA) physical status classification replaced the number of discharge diagnoses as the second factor. An ASA score of three or greater garners one point in the NNIS system. Duration of the operation is the third factor, and is worth one point if the procedure lasts longer than 75% of similar procedures. A patient's risk for surgical site infection can therefore be stratified as NNIS class 0, 1, 2, or 3, based on which of the three risk factors the patient has. Although the risk of infection increases within the wound classification, it has been shown to be also dependent within each wound class on the NNIS classification (Table 1) (11).

The type of organism encountered in a SSI depends on the type of surgery performed; gram-positive organisms are more likely to be encountered in clean cases, whereas gram-negative organisms are more likely to be encountered in clean contaminated cases involving the alimentary tract. The most prevalent pathogen isolated from SSIs is *S. aureus*. The prevalence of *S. aureus* as a pathogen in surgical infections has remained constant, whereas the proportion of isolates identified as MRSA has continued to increase. According to reports from the Sentry Antimicrobial Surveillance Program from the United States and Canada in 2000, MRSA is responsible for 30% of SSIs compared to 24% three years earlier (4,12). Increased rates of MRSA infections are of particular

TABLE 1 Surgical Site Infection Rates by Wound Class Versus National Nosocomial Infection Surveillance Class

Wound class	All (%)	NNIS 0 (%)	NNIS 1 (%)	NNIS 2 (%)	NNIS 3 (%)
Clean	2.1	1.0	2.3	5.4	N/A
Clean contaminated	3.3	2.1	4.0	9.5	N/A
Contaminated	6.4	N/A	3.4	6.8	13.2
Dirty/infected	7.1	N/A	3.1	8.1	12.8
All	2.8	1.5	2.9	6.8	13.0

Source: From Ref. 9.

concern because patients infected with this pathogen have higher mortality rates, greater morbidity, and utilize more health care resources compared with those who have infections caused by methicillin-susceptible pathogens (13,14).

Successful therapy of these infections depends on the early suspicion and identification of resistant pathogens and subsequent use of antibiotics against MRSA.

Prophylaxis for surgical site infection is a well-established practice and the target of performance improvement in the United States. Surgical site prophylaxis for many clean surgical cases uses drugs that have been effective against MSSA. The explosion of MRSA, whether it is CA-MRSA or HA-MRSA, has produced a dilemma. Prophylaxis for MRSA SSI remains a source of controversy; however, as delineated by the CDC, patients at a high risk for MRSA should undergo prophylaxis with an anti-MRSA agent (15). Mupirocin treatment of *S. aureus*–colonized patients prior to surgery has not been shown to decrease the incidence of surgical site infection (16). No guidelines exist about the decolonization of patients prior to surgery; as part of infection control measures, decolonization of patients detected to be MRSA colonized has been practiced in certain hospitals (17).

Blistering Distal Dactylitis

Blistering distal dactylitis (BDD) is a distinct clinical entity involving localized infection of the volar fat pad of the distal phalanx of the fingers and sometimes toes. If left untreated, it can lead to progression and distal digit amputation. It should be differentiated from bullous impetigo, which has the same etiology but is more superficial (Fig. 1).

The characteristic clinical appearance is fluid-filled blisters containing thin, white pus. The BDD is typically seen in children between the ages of 2 and 16 years, although it has also been reported in infants and adults.

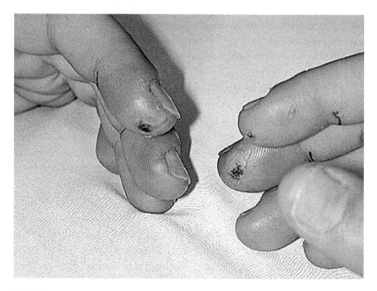

FIGURE 1 Blistering distal dactylitis. *Source*: From Ref. 18.

Autoinoculation of the finger from nose picking is one proposed course. The BDD is usually associated with group A β-hemolytic *Streptococcus*, but can also be caused by *S. aureus* and *S. epidermidis*. Multiple-finger involvement may be a predictor of *S. aureus* infection. Increasing reports of MRSA BDD is being reported, necessitating appropriate antibiotic coverage for this organism (18).

MANAGEMENT OF COMPLICATED SKIN AND SOFT TISSUE INFECTIONS

The management of cSSTI is based on two important considerations: (*i*) the host risk factors and (*ii*) the systemic host response to the infection. On the basis of these two considerations, a management algorithm was developed and is shown in Figure 2.

The host risk factors well established for SSI are multiple and include increasing age, poor nutritional status, uncontrolled diabetes, impaired immunity, obesity, and poor tissue oxygenation at the site of incision. Less important risk factors include nicotine use, prior hospitalization, and other infections at a remote site from the site in question. In addition to environmental factors in the operating room and surgical technique, these lesser factors are important risk factors for surgical site infection and other cSSTI (19).

Systemic host response is manifested by increasing temperature and WBC; great caution needs to be applied in the elderly, the very young, and the immunocompromised, as the systemic responses could be attenuated, manifesting only as a low grade temperature, hypothermia, a left shift, leucopenia, systemic sepsis, or local symptoms only.

Expectant therapy alone for cSSTI is not an option. An important component of therapy even in uncomplicated SSTI is incision and drainage (2). The addition of systemic antibiotics for uncomplicated SSTI remains the subject of debate (20). A randomized double-blind trial comparing placebo to cephalexin in 166 patients undergoing drainage of uncomplicated abscesses provides the strongest evidence yet that antibiotics are not

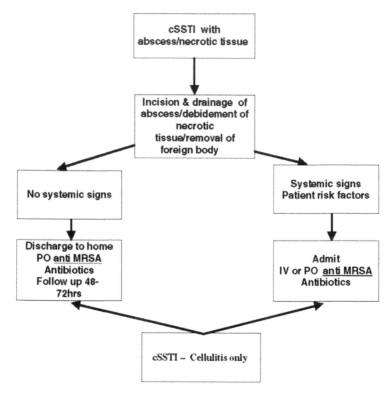

FIGURE 2 Management of MRSA-complicated skin and soft tissue infections.

needed. A total of 68% of cultures yielded *S. aureus* strains, 88% of which were MRSA and 94% of the MRSA strains were positive for Panton-Valentine leukocidin. In all 90.5% of placebo, recipients had a clinical cure as compared with 84.1% of cephalexin recipients (21).

Surgical intervention being the mainstay of therapy consists of incision and drainage of abscesses and debridement of all necrotic tissue, and removal of any foreign bodies. The only exception is cellulitis. Caution has to be exercised with cellulitis. Cellulitis may be appropriately treated with antibiotics alone, but unresolving cellulitis with appropriate antibiotic therapy should prompt an evaluation for a deep abscess or underlying fasciitis. Removal of foreign bodies, including suture material, artificial mesh, and prosthetics, is important. Foreign bodies serve as a nidus for bacteria and are associated with biofilm formation and bacterial deposition, which facilitates persistence of infection. The biofilm around the foreign body also prevents antibiotics from reaching the bacteria. After incision/drainage and debridement, wounds should be left open and loosely packed with a saline-soaked gauze and covered with a dry dressing. The dressing is changed at least twice a day and allowed to granulate and heal secondarily. In cases where necrotic tissue and debris are present, repeat sharp debridement should be performed; in addition, the saline soaked gauze dressing can be substituted with a 0.5% sodium hypochlorite solution (Dakin's solution)–soaked gauze or placement of papain/urea ointment (Accuzyme®) for chemical debridement. Alternatively, in large clean wounds a vacuum-assisted closure device may speed the healing process.

Antibiotic therapy is usually an adjuvant to surgical therapy. In patients with MRSA risk factors, systemic manifestations, or deep tissue infections, antibiotics should be administered. Whether antibiotics are given orally or intravenously is dependent on the extent of infection, presence or absence of systemic symptoms, and the availability of an oral antibiotic that will effectively cover suspected or proven organisms (Fig. 2). Hospitalization is usually determined by the patient's overall clinical status and whether the patient needs intravenous antibiotics. Outpatient intravenous antibiotics are an option if no oral counterpart is available and the patient's clinical status permits.

Poor response to therapy manifesting as persistence of local or systemic symptoms implies inadequate source control, poor drainage of an abscess, or resistance of the bacteria to chosen antibiotics.

Debridement of remaining or new necrotic tissue should be performed as well as a search for undrained abscesses done through ultrasonography or computed tomography. Osteomyelitis should always be suspected in patients with diabetic foot infections. If the site of infection is clean and no other source of infection is located, appropriate tissue cultures should be obtained, and when MRSA is cultured, administration of a different antibiotic with MRSA activity and different mechanism of action or better tissue penetration should be administered.

The length of antibiotic therapy in cSSTI has not been studied. It is my belief that the duration of antibiotic therapy is dependent on resolution of local and systemic symptoms rather than on a specific number of days. In young, healthy individuals, antibiotics can be stopped as soon as local and systemic symptoms have resolved. This should also be considered in patients with risk factors, although greater caution should be exercised, especially if the host is immunocompromised. Antibiotics should be used for longer periods in patients with diabetic foot infections and patients with osteomyelitis. The duration of treatment remains controversial and is dependent on the extent of bone debridement and vascular disease, and improvement in local signs (22).

Most of these patients had additional systemic antibiotics withheld or treatment with an antibiotic to which the bacterium was not susceptible. These treatment failures have two characteristics: treatment with a single systemic antibiotic or treatment with an antibiotic to which the bacterium was not susceptible (2). These observations have skewed opinions toward early or empiric MRSA adjuvant antibiotic coverage in patients undergoing incisions and drainage of SSTI (20).

CHOICE OF ANTIBIOTICS IN MRSA-COMPLICATED SSTI

Because MRSA infection rates continue to increase, both in the hospital and the community, resistance needs to be considered when designing a treatment regimen for cSSTI. Factors that determine success or failure of an antimicrobial agent in treating a specific infection include the site of infection and the spectrum of activity, efficacy, and safety profile (23). Both patient factors and prevalence of MRSA influence the choice of empirical antibiotics. Individual risk factors need to be considered in addition to the prevalence of MRSA within a particular institution or population group. Some facilities use a tool to predict the probability of methicillin resistance in patients with a suspected *S. aureus* infection (24,25). If CA-MRSA is strongly suspected on the basis of local prevalence data or epidemiological and/or clinical clues, coverage for that organism becomes essential. Appropriate outpatient treatment can be given with trimethoprim-sulfamethoxazole (TMP-SMX), minocycline, doxycycline, or clindamycin. Numerous treatment failures have been attributed to inducible clindamycin resistance: any erythromycin-resistant but clindamycin-susceptible strain may harbor inducible resistance (26). None of these drugs is FDA approved for MRSA cSSTI, and none have undergone rigorous evaluation in clinical trials. In addition, no randomized prospective data are available to support one oral agent over another in this setting. However, the availability, low cost, and long-standing use of these drugs in clinical practice have given them a de facto acceptance for the treatment of MRSA cSSTI.

Newer fluoroquinolones (e.g., gatifloxacin, moxifloxacin, and levofloxacin) have enhanced activity against *Staphylococcus*, and combined with rifampin, appear effective in diverse clinical scenarios (27). Increasing fluoroquinolone resistance among CA-MRSA, some of the gram-negative bacilli, and the association of fluoroquinolones with *Clostridium difficile* colitis suggest that fluoroquinolones should not be first-line agents for empirical treatment (28).

Several other antimicrobials are available for the treatment of MRSA cSSTI. Vancomycin has been the treatment of choice for infections caused by MRSA; however, current data indicate that it may not be the optimal choice in cSSTI. Thirty years after vancomycin became available, vancomycin-resistant *Enterococcus* (VRE) was first identified in France in

1986. Of great concern was the emergence of reduced vancomycin susceptibility in *S. aureus*, which many feared to be a prelude to full resistance. In a single-institution study of SSTI, the minimal inhibitory concentration (MIC) was less than or equal to 0.5 in 100% of MRSA in 2003; in 2006 only 60.5% of MRSA had an MIC ≤ 0.5 with 31% having an MIC $= 2$ (29). A higher MIC of vancomycin has been shown to be associated with increased failure of vancomycin therapy (30).

Several new antimicrobials against MRSA have received FDA approval for treating MRSA cSSTI. Linezolid, daptomycin, and tigecycline have been approved for use in MRSA cSSTI; quinupristin/dalfopristin was approved for cSSTI, but not cSSTI due to MRSA.

A large prospective, randomized, multinational trial compared linezolid with vancomycin or a semisynthetic penicillin in 1200 patients with cSSTI. Clinical cure was achieved in 92.2% and 88.5% of patients treated with linezolid and vancomycin, respectively ($p = 0.057$). A total of 134 patients with MRSA cSSTI were found in both the linezolid and vancomycin group. Patient outcome with MRSA infections was better when treated with linezolid (88.6% cure) than when treated with vancomycin (66.9% cure) ($p < 0.001$) (31). A subset analysis from this trial compared 66 SSI patients receiving linezolid with 69 SSI patients receiving vancomycin for clinical and microbiologic cure. Among patients with MRSA infections, clinical cure in both groups was similar, but microbiologic eradication of the bacteria from the wound was achieved in 87% of the SSI patients treated with linezolid versus 48% treated with vancomycin ($p = 0.0022$) (32). Linezolid is the only agent with available pharmacoeconomic data. Though it has a high acquisition cost, it is 100% bioavailable when administered orally, and markedly reduces the length of intravenous therapy. Reduction in intravenous therapy was almost 11 days in patients with MRSA infections (1.8 total intravenous days for linezolid compared to 12.6 days of intravenous therapy for vancomycin), and by seven days overall. Length of stay was decreased by at least two days when infections caused by methicillin-sensitive or methicillin-resistant organisms were treated with linezolid (33). Incremental analysis of total costs and cure showed that linezolid resulted in a mean 5.7% increase in clinical cure rate concomitant with a mean $652 in cost saving per patient treated for cSSTI in the intent to treat population (34). A more recent study comparing linezolid to vancomycin in MRSA confirmed cSSTI where vancomycin was dosed to 15 mg/kg with dose adjustment based on creatinine clearance and trough levels revealed that the cure rate with linezolid was comparable to vancomycin (35).

Daptomycin was compared with vancomycin or semisynthetic penicillin in a phase 3, multicenter, double-blind study consisting of 562 patients with cSSTI. Clinical cure of 81% was observed in both groups. Microbiologic eradication was achieved in 91% of patients treated with daptomycin versus 92% of patients treated with comparators (36).

Tigecycline is a novel glycopeptide that displays expanded broad-spectrum activity against gram-positive cocci, including MRSA and VRE, gram-negative bacilli, atypical organisms, and anaerobes. Clinical trials of tigecycline for cSSTI have demonstrated equivalent efficacy to vancomycin and suggest that it will be a reasonable alternative for multidrug-resistant organisms (37). The broad-spectrum activity of tige-cycline makes it an agent for consideration in patients with cSSTI secondary to multiple organisms often seen in patients with perirectal abscesses and necrotizing fasciitis.

Several novel antimicrobials with activity against MRSA cSSTI are currently awaiting FDA clearance or in late phase 3 trials and include dalbavancin, oritavancin, televancin, ceftobiprole, iclaprim, and ceftaro-line. Longer half-lives with more convenient dosing schedules and different mechanisms of action are possible advantages of some of these newer agents.

The choice of any of these newer FDA-approved agents as opposed to the older agents that show activity against CA-MRSA is not easy. The clinician must consider the likelihood of CA-MRSA versus HA-MRSA, patient drug allergies, drug interactions, pharmacokinetics, available oral therapy for outpatient use, pharmacoeconomic data, and the emergence of resistant organisms in the future with widespread utilization. As with the treatment of ventilator-associated pneumonia, new evidence in the treatment of cSSTI reveals that early appropriate antibiotic therapy is crucial. Failure of appropriate antibiotic therapy can increase mortality, length of stay, and costs (38). Similarly, delayed appropriate therapy can increase length of stay and total costs (39). In the treatment of cSSTI, it is therefore important to follow the guideline provided in Figure 2 for adjuvant antibiotic administration and to choose the most appropriate empiric antibiotic on the basis of local epidemiological data and until final cultures are available.

REFERENCES

1. Uncomplicated and complicated skin and skin structure infections—developing antimicrobial drugs for treatment: Guidance for industry. Available at: www.fda.gov/cder/guidance/2566dfr.pdf 7-22-1998. Last accessed August 12, 2006.
2. Cohen PR. Community acquired methicillin-resistant *Staphylococcus aureus* skin infections: a review of epidemiology, clinical features, management and prevention. Int J Dermatol 2007; 46:1–11.
3. Moet GJ, Jones RN, Biedenbach DJ, et al. Contemporary causes of skin and soft tissue infections in North America, Latin America, and Europe: report from the SENTRY Antimicrobial Surveillance Program (1998–2004). Diagn Microbiol Infect Dis 2007; 57(1):7–13.
4. Rennie RP, Jones RN, Mutnick AH; SENTRY Program Study Group (North America). Occurrence and antimicrobial susceptibility patterns of pathogens isolated from skin and soft tissue infections: report from the SENTRY Antimicrobial Surveillance Program (United States and Canada, 2000). Diagn Microbiol Infect Dis 2003; 45(4):287–293.
5. Naimi TS, LeDell KH, Como-Sabetti K, et al. Comparison of community- and health care-associated methicillin-resistant *Staphylococcus aureus* infection. J Am Med Assoc 2003; 290(22):2976–2984.
6. Weber JT. Community-associated methicillin-resistant *Staphylococcus aureus*. Clin Infect Dis 2005; 41(suppl 4):S269–S272.

7. Baggett HC, Hennessy TW, Rudolph K, et al. Community-onset methicillin-resistant *Staphylococcus aureus* associated with antibiotic use and the cytotoxin Panton-Valentine leukocidin during a furunculosis outbreak in rural Alaska. J Infect Dis 2004; 189(9):1565–1573.

8. Miller LG, Perdreau-Remmington F, Rieg G, et al. Necrotizing fasciitis caused by community-associated methicillin-resistant *Staphylococcus aureus* in Los Angeles. N Engl J Med 2005; 352:1445–1453.

9. Horan TC, Gaynes RP, Martone WJ, et al. CDC definitions of nosocomial surgical site infections. Infect Control Hosp Epidemiol 1992; 13:606–608.

10. Culver DH, Horan TC, Gaynes RP, et al. Surgical wound infection rates by wound class, operative procedure, and patient risk index. Am J Med 1991; 91(suppl 3B):152–157.

11. Knight R, Charbonneau P, Ratzer E, et al. Prophylactic antibiotics are not indicated in clean general surgery cases. Am J Surg 2001; 182:682–686.

12. Doern GV, Jones RN, Pfaller MA, et al. and the SENTRY study group (North America). Bacterial pathogens isolated from patients with skin and soft tissue infections: frequency of occurrence and antimicrobial susceptibility patterns from the SENTRY Antimicrobial Surveillance Program (United States and Canada, 1997). Diagn Microbiol Infect Dis 1999; 34:65–72.

13. Kaye KS, Engemann JJ, Mozaffari E, et al. Reference group choice and antibiotic resistance outcomes. Emerg Infect Dis 2004; 10(6):1125–1128.

14. Engemann JJ, Carmeli Y, Cosgrove SE, et al. Adverse clinical and economic outcomes attributable to methicillin resistance among patients with *Staphylococcus aureus* surgical site infection. Clin Infect Dis 2003; 36(5):592–598.

15. Bratzler DW, Houck PM; Surgical Infection Prevention Guidelines Writers Workgroup. Antimicrobial prophylaxis for surgery: an advisory statement from the National Surgical Infection Prevention Project. Clin Infect Dis 2004; 38(12):1706.

16. Perl TM, Cullen JJ, Wenzel RP, et al. Intranasal mupirocin to prevent postoperative *Staphylococcus aureus* infection. N Engl J Med 2002; 346(24): 1871–1877.

17. Rao N, Jacobs S, Joyce L. Cost-effective eradication of an outbreak of methicillin-resistant *Staphylococcus aureus* in a community teaching hospital. Infect Control Hosp Epidemiol 1988; 9(6):255–260.

18. Mangram AJ, Horan TC, Pearson ML, et al. Guideline for prevention of surgical site infection, 1999. Hospital Infection Control Practices Advisory Committee. Infect Control Hosp Epidemiol 1999; 20(4):250–278.

19. Huh SY, Daya M. Dermatology quiz. Resident and Staff Physician 2006; 852(6):37–38.

20. Hammond SP, Baden LR. Clinical decisions. Management of skin and soft tissue infection—polling results. N Engl J Med 2008; 359(15):e20:1–5.

21. Rajendran PM, Young D, Maurer T, et al. Randomized, double-blind, placebo-controlled trial of cephalexin for treatment of uncomplicated skin abscesses in a population at risk for community-acquired methicillin-resistant *Staphylococcus aureus* infection. Antimicrob Agents Chemother 2007; 51(11):4044–4048.

22. Lipsky BA, Berendt AR, Deery HG, et al. Diagnosis and treatment of diabetic foot infections. Clin Infect Dis 2004; 39(7):885–910.

23. Stevens DL. The relevance of antibiotic tissue penetration for treating complicated skin and soft tissue infections caused by methicillin-resistant *Staphylococcus aureus*: an evidence-based review. Med Ed Direct 2004; 4:1–6.

24. Rezende NA, Blumberg HM, Metzger BS, et al. Risk factors for methicillin resistance among patients with *Staphylococcus aureus* bacteremia at the time of hospital admission. Am J Med Sci 2002; 323:117–123.

25. Lodise TP Jr., McKinnon PS, Rybak M. Prediction model to identify patients with *Staphylococcus aureus* bacteremia at risk of methicillin resistance. Infect Control Hosp Epidemiol 2003; 24:655–661.

26. Siberry GK, Tekle T, Carroll K, et al. Failure of clindamycin treatment of methicillin-resistant *Staphylococcus aureus* expressing inducible clindamycin resistance in vitro. Clin Infect Dis 2003; 37:1257–1260.

27. Schrenzel J, Harbarth S, Schockmel G, et al. Swiss Staphylococcal Study Group. A randomized clinical trial to compare fleroxacin-rifampicin with flucloxacillin or vancomycin for the treatment of staphylococcal infection. Clin Infect Dis 2004; 39:1285–1292.

28. Itani KMF. Infections in the surgical patient: an update on trends and treatments. Am J Surg 2003; 186(5A):1S–3S.

29. Awad SS, Elhabash SI, Lee L, et al. Increasing incidence of methicillin-resistant *Staphylococcus aureus* skin and soft-tissue infections: reconsideration of empiric antimicrobial therapy. Am J Surg 2007; 194(5):606–610.

30. Sakoulas G, Moise-Broder PA, Schentag J, et al. Relationship of MIC and bactericidal activity to efficacy of vancomycin for treatment of methicillin-resistant *Staphylococcus aureus* bacteremia. J Clin Microbiol 2004; 42(6):2398–2402.

31. Weigelt JA, Itani KMF, Stevens D, et al. Linezolid vs vancomycin in the treatment of complicated skin and soft tissue infections. Antimicrob Agents Chemother 2005; 49(6):1–7.

32. Weigelt J, Kaafarani HMA, Itani KMF, et al. Linezolid eradicates MRSA better than vancomycin from surgical-site infections. Am J Surg 2004; 188:760–766.

33. Itani KMF, Weigelt J, Li JZ, et al. Linezolid reduces length of stay and intravenous therapy duration compared with vancomycin for complicated skin and soft tissue infections due to suspected methicillin resistant *Staphylococcus aureus*. Int J Antimicrob Agents 2005; 26(6):442–448.

34. Mc Kinnon PS, Sorensen S, Liu L, et al. The impact of linezolid on economic outcomes and determinants of cost in patients with documented or suspected MRSA complicated skin and soft-tissue infections. Ann Pharmacother 2006; 40(6):1017–1023.

35. Itani KMF, Weigelt J, Stevens DL, et al. Efficacite et tolerance du linezolide (LZD) versus vancomycine (VAN) dans le traitement des infections compliquees de la peau et des tissues mous (ICPTM) documentees a SARM (abstract). Med Mal Infect 2009; 39:S8–S9.

36. Arbeit RD, Maki D, Tally FP, et al.; Daptomycin 98-01 and 99-01 Investigators. The safety and efficacy of daptomycin for the treatment of complicated skin and skin-structure infections. Clin Infect Dis 2004; 38:1673–1681.

37. Breedt J, Teras J, Gardovskis J, et al.; Tigecycline 305 cSSSI Study Group. Safety and efficacy of tigecycline in treatment of skin and skin structure infections: results of a double-blind phase 3 comparison study with vancomycin–aztreonam. Antimicrob Agents Chemother 2005; 49(11):4658–4666.

38. delsberg J, Berger A, Weber DJ, et al. Clinical and economic consequences of failure of initial antibiotic therapy for hospitalized patients with complicated skin and skin-structure infections. Infect Control Hosp Epidemiol 2008; 29(2):160–169.

39. Itani KMF, Akhras KS, Stellhorn R, et al. Outcomes associated with initial vs. later vancomycin use to cover for methicillin-resistant *Staphylococcus aureus* in patients with skin and soft tissue infections. Pharmacoeconomics 2009; 27(5):421–430.

MRSA in the Diabetic Foot

Lee C. Rogers and Nicholas J. Bevilacqua
Amputation Prevention Center, Valley Presbyterian Hospital, Los Angeles,
California, U.S.A.

David G. Armstrong
Department of Surgery, University of Arizona College of Medicine, Tucson,
Arizona, U.S.A.

DIABETIC FOOT: THE SCOPE OF THE PROBLEM

Diabetic foot problems are a major burden on health care resources and
come at great costs. Diabetic foot ulcers (DFUs) will affect up to 25% of
people with diabetes during their lifetime. DFUs/diabetic foot infections
(DFIs) are the most common reason for hospitalization among diabetic
patients in the United States (1). Hospital length of stay is 59% longer for
diabetic patients with ulcers when compared to those without ulcers (2).
Foot ulcers and amputations were estimated to cost the U.S. health care
system $30 billion in 2007 (3). Foot ulcers are the antecedent event in
84% of diabetic lower extremity amputations (LEAs) (4). More than half
of the approximately 120,000 nontraumatic amputations performed each
year are on people with diabetes, making diabetes the leading cause of
nontraumatic amputations (5). The Centers for Disease Control 1999
Surveillance Summary for nontraumatic amputations revealed that LEAs
increased by 24% between 1983 and 1996. There were 10.2 LEAs per
1000 diabetic patients (6). Infection precedes 59% of diabetic amputations
(4). A person with diabetes and one LEA has a 50% chance of developing a
limb-threatening condition on the contralateral limb within two years (7).
Diabetics with foot problems are at increased risk of morbidity and
mortality. Jeffcoate et al. followed 449 diabetic patients with ulcers for

12 months. Only 45.0% were alive, without amputation, and ulcer free at the endpoint. A total of 11% of patients had undergone some form of amputation and 17% had died (8). Ramsey et al. reviewed 8905 patients with diabetes; the cumulative three-year survival rate was 72% for patients with a foot ulcer versus 87% for those without ulcers (9).

Lavery et al. followed 1666 patients with diabetes for an average of 27 months. Ulcerations developed in 247 patients and infections in 151 patients, with an infection to ulcer ratio of 0.56 (10). The diagnosis of DFI is primarily based on the clinical examination. Diagnosis can be made by the presence of purulence or two or more of the following signs/symptoms: erythema, induration, pain, tenderness, or warmth (11). Laboratory testing should not be relied upon to diagnose or rule out foot infection in diabetic patients. Leukocytosis is only present in 46% of diabetic patients with moderate to severe DFIs (12). People with diabetes have blunted immune responses because of abnormalities in granulocyte adherence, chemotaxis, and phagocytosis. Plasma glucose levels greater than 220 mg/dL in diabetics on day 1 after surgery is associated with a 30% postoperative infection rate (13). O'Meara et al. conducted a systematic review of methods used to diagnose DFI (14). They concluded that it was not possible to describe the optimal methods of diagnosing infection in diabetic patients with foot ulceration with the evidence identified in their systematic review.

While an optimal method may still be elusive, a number of attempts at establishing methods for the diagnosis and management of DFI are available. The Infectious Disease Society of America (IDSA) has published guidelines for diagnosing DFI as well as a classification for presence and extent of infection (15). The IDSA divided infections into four categories of severity on the basis of clinical manifestations: uninfected, mild, moderate, or severe infections. This system was later validated and correlates with the incidence of hospitalization and amputation (Table 1) (17). Another commonly used simple classification is non-limb-threatening or limb-threatening DFI (18). Non-limb-threatening infections have less than 2 cm of

TABLE 1 The Infectious Diseases Society of America Classification of Diabetic Foot Wounds and Related Complications

IDSA class	Description	Complications
Mild infection (non-limb-threatening)	<2 cm surrounding cellulites, no deep spread, no systemic signs	Hospitalization (11%) Amputation (4%)
Moderate infection (limb-threatening)	>2 cm surrounding cellulites and/or deep spread to fascia, tendon, muscle, or bone. No systemic signs	Hospitalization (54%) Amputation (47%)
Severe infection (limb- and life-threatening)	Moderate infection with systemic signs of infection, such as SIRS or sepsis	Hospitalization (89%) Amputation (78%)

Abbreviation: IDSA, Infectious Diseases Society of America; SIRS, systemic inflammatory response syndrome.
Source: From Ref. 16.

surrounding cellulitis, whereas limb-threatening infections have more extensive cellulitis. The University of Texas Diabetic Foot Ulcer Classification scheme is a useful tool to classify DFU on the basis of depth, presence/absence of infection, and ischemia (19). Although not a direct classification of DFI, per se, it is highly prognostic for amputation (20).

The diagnosis of osteomyelitis (OM) in DFIs is difficult and many times a controversial topic between clinicians. Grayson et al. reported that palpating bone with a sterile blunt metal instrument inserted into a wound had a positive predictive value of 89% for OM (21). However, their study population were patients enrolled in an antibiotic trial for limb-threatening DFIs, meaning these patients already had a high pretest probability of OM. This may have lead to the overrepresentation of OM in their study (22). El Maghraby and colleagues published a thorough review on the accuracy of a variety of imaging modalities that exist to diagnose OM

(23). They reported that plain radiographs have a sensitivity and specificity of 43% to 75% and 75% to 83%, respectively. Scintigraphic methods were reviewed and Tech[99] triphasic bone scans had a sensitivity of 73% to 100%. Tech[99] scans are not very specific and can be "hot" (positive) with any number of bone pathologies, such as fracture, postsurgical osteotomies, tumors, periosteal inflammation/bruising, or Charcot foot. Galium[67] citrate scans were more specific for infection with a specificity as high as 92%. White blood cell–labeled bone scans (In[111] or HMPAO) had sensitivities and specificities in the range of 80% to 90%. MRI had a sensitivity/specificity for OM as high as 100%/96%. Difficulty is encountered when attempting to use MRI to diagnose OM of the smaller bones in the foot (e.g., toes); thus, an extremity coil is recommended.

Appropriate antibiotic therapy of a DFI usually requires culturing the wound and performing sensitivity testing on isolated pathogens (24,25). However, a wound culture is not to be used to diagnose wound infection, but rather to direct the therapy. Emphasis on a proper wound culture technique is paramount. Uninfected wounds should not be cultured. The accuracy of a wound culture depends on obtaining an appropriate specimen (24). There are several different techniques used for obtaining tissue samples from the wound. Some methods are superficial swab cultures, needle aspiration, and wound biopsy. Superficial swab cultures are often used in the clinical setting, as some believe that they are cost effective, less invasive, and adequately diagnostic (25). There is inconsistency in the literature whether a superficial swab culture reflects surface flora only or the causative pathogens (26–28). A proper wound culture should be obtained after debridement of all infected and necrotic tissue. This requires careful attention to sterile technique as well as selection of the optimal portion of the wound for sampling (25,29). Deep, initially unexposed tissue removed with sterile instruments will generally yield the most accurate culture results (30). It is important to obtain both aerobic and anaerobic cultures of the wound. Once the cultures are sent, antibiotic therapy patient should empirically be started on patients.

The microbiology of DFIs generally depends on the severity of the infection. Non-limb-threatening infections are usually the result of gram-positive bacteria, predominately *Staphylococcus aureus* and *Streptococcus* spp. (31). Limb-threatening infections tend to be polymicrobial with a mixture of gram-positive, gram-negative, aerobic, and anaerobic bacteria. An average of 2.8 to 5.8 bacteria are cultured from these infections (11,32,33).

MRSA IN DFIS

Previous reports found up to 30% of skin isolates were methicillin-resistant *Staphylococcus aureus* (MRSA) (34). Tentolouris et al. looked at MRSA prevalence in infected and uninfected DFUs. *S. aureus* was the most common pathogen of which almost 50% were methicillin resistant (35). Dang et al. evaluated wound swab cultures in 63 outpatients with diabetes and foot ulcers and found that gram-positive bacteria predominated in 84.2% (*S. aureus* in 79%) (36). MRSA was found in 30.2%, which is almost twice as that reported in a similar study only three years earlier (37). Similarly, in 911 patients with chronic ulcers, Roghmann found that 30% were colonized with MRSA (38).

Risk factors for MRSA infections include recent previous hospitalization (39–41), nursing home residence (41,42), and prior antibiotic usage (42,43), but perhaps the single most important risk factor is a previous history of MRSA infection/colonization (42–44). Of the 209 patients studied by Huang et al., an 18-month risk of reinfection with MRSA was detected in 29%. Twenty-eight percent of those infections involved bacteremia and 56% involved pneumonia, soft tissue, OM, or septic arthritis (44). Risk factors for MRSA infection in orthopedic and burn patient admissions were previous hospital stay within three months, the use of broad-spectrum antibiotics in the past two weeks, and previous infection/carriage of MRSA. Sixty-two percent of the patients with a previous history of MRSA developed reinfection (43).

As a result of immunopathy, people with diabetes have increased morbidity and mortality from MRSA infections. Diabetes is associated with persistent bacteremia in patients with MRSA (45). Patients whose wounds are colonized with MRSA have a risk ratio of 16 for developing MRSA bacteremia (38). MRSA bacteremia is associated with a 43% mortality rate compared with 20% for MSSA bacteremia (46). Tsao et al. studied infected diabetic and nondiabetic mice with MSSA and MRSA. Diabetic mice infected with MRSA died at an average of 10.6 ($\pm$0.7) days whereas non-diabetic mice infected with MRSA died at 19.1 ($\pm$1.4) days. MSSA infections did not cause death in either group of mice. Diabetic mice infected with MRSA had significant increase in C-reactive protein, fibrinogen, fibronectin, and von Willebrand factor compared to nondiabetic mice. The authors concluded that MRSA infections in diabetic mice accelerated the inflammatory process, endothelial injury, and blood coagulation, ultimately leading to a quicker death (47). Additionally, there are case reports of MRSA causing necrotizing fasciitis in patients with diabetes (48,49).

Diabetic outcomes are worse in patients with MRSA infections, and length of hospital stay is longer for these patients (38). Grimble et al. (50) reviewed 30 patients undergoing major amputation. Seventeen of 30 amputated limbs had cultures positive for MRSA. Mortality was 43% in patients with MRSA-infected limbs compared with only 9% in non-MRSA infections. Primary healing was achieved in only 4 of 17 (24%) amputations with MRSA infections. Richards and coworkers (51) prospectively followed 25 patients with 33 primary amputations (14 above the knee and 19 below the knee). At the time of surgery, 45% of the legs were colonized or infected with MRSA. Postoperative stump infection developed in 24% of patients, 71% of which were MRSA infections.

CLINICAL APPROACH TO TREATMENT OF DFIS AND ULCERS

Adequate debridement is perhaps the most important initial treatment of diabetic wound infections. Devitalized tissue in a wound can delay healing, predispose to infection, and interfere with adequate assessment

(52–54). Debridement is removing necrotic tissue, foreign material, and infecting bacteria from a wound (55). The goal is to excise the wound completely until only normal, soft, and well-vascularized tissue remains (55). Debridement in an operating room is usually necessary for limb-threatening infections, whereas clinic debridement can be performed in non-limb-threatening infections. The wound is debrided until only healthy, bleeding tissue is present. The role of debridement is to convert an infected fibrotic wound to a healthy granular wound.

Over the past decade, there have been numerous biotechnological advances in wound healing modalities, including the development of acellular matrix–based materials, cytokines, and bioengineered tissue replacements. All of these advanced technologies are only helpful when the wound is uninfected and well vascularized with granular tissue. The role of these modalities is to enhance granulation tissue and ultimately ease the transition to wound closure by secondary intention, delayed primary closure, or skin grafting.

The use of negative pressure wound therapy (NPWT) with the WOUND V.A.C.® (Kinetic Concepts, Inc., San Antonio, Texas) or other NPWT devices is, in large part, responsible for simplifying wound care because it helps promote granulation tissue formation so that the wound area and depth becomes manageable (55). NPWT applies localized negative pressure to help uniformly draw wounds closed. It has cellular microdeformational effects that help remove interstitial fluid and infectious material. The V.A.C. provides a closed, moist wound healing environment and helps promote flap and graft survival (56). A multi-center, randomized controlled trial compared NPWT to standard moist wound care after partial diabetic foot amputation. The rate of wound healing and granulation tissue formation was faster in the NPWT group compared to the controls. Both groups had similar frequency and severity of adverse events (57).

Cell-based technologies help deliver exogenous growth factors to the wound bed. Two FDA-approved products are Apligraf® and

Dermagraft®. Extracellular matrix scaffolds help organize the healing process and provide a scaffolding for the host cells to grow. These include Graftjacket® Matrix, Integra® BMD, Oasis® (non-cross-linked xenograft) and Gammagraft™ (irradiated cadaveric skin). Isolated recombinant growth factors, like platelet-derived growth factor in Regranex®, can be used to promote granulation tissue.

Offloading is key in the treatment of DFUs. A vascularized, uninfected, granular wound will not heal unless the mechanical forces are reduced or eliminated. There are many offloading modalities currently in use today. Some examples are bed rest, wheel chair, crutches, total contact casts (TCCs), removable cast walkers (RCWs), instant total contact cast (iTCC), half shoes, custom splints, and therapeutic shoes. Crutches are not advocated since diabetics with peripheral diseases have other central diseases and crutch walking increases the energy of ambulation. These patients may not have adequate cardiac reserves for ambulating with crutches. In addition, diabetics with peripheral neuropathy have sensory ataxia and may risk falling while attempting to use crutches. A Roll-A-Bout® (Roll-A-Bout Corp., Federica, Maryland) is a "rolling crutch" that allows offloading of the foot while the healthy extremity propels the device and may be useful in these patients. Wheelchairs are also effective pressure reduction devices; however, most patients' homes are not designed to accommodate the bulkiness of the wheelchairs and this can lead to high levels of noncompliant activity (58).

The TCC is effective because it permits walking while offloading by transferring some weight to the cylindrical calf and uniformly distributing the remaining pressures over the entire plantar surface of the foot (59,60). However, applying the TCC is technically demanding and requires training and experience. Because improper cast application can cause skin irritation and in some cases even frank ulceration, this can be its single biggest negative feature. RCWs offer several potential advantages over the traditional TCC. Gait lab studies suggest that the amount of pressure reduction for certain RCWs is equivalent to that of TCCs (61).

Unfortunately, they are removable, which is their greatest drawback as patients do not use them during all ambulatory activities. One study found that patients only wore their removable offloading device for less than 30% of their total daily activity (62). Armstrong et al. suggested a potential alternative, an RCW made less removable. This simple concept, termed as "instant total contact cast" (63), involves simply wrapping the RCW with either a layer of cohesive bandage or plaster/fiberglass, thereby making it more difficult for patients to remove. The iTCC then may have the benefit of adequate offloading (on par with the TCC) as well as "forced adherence" to the prescribed course of pressure reduction.

MODIFICATION OF ANTIMICROBIAL TREATMENT IN THE ERA OF MRSA

Initial empiric therapy of non-limb-threatening infections, being primarily gram-positive, consists of oral outpatient therapy utilizing medications such as cephalexin, amoxicillin/clavulanate, or clindamycin. More severe limb-threatening infections are treated with inpatient intraveneous therapies including piperacillin/tazobactam (64), ertapenem (65) imipenem, or a fluorquinolone. Upon review of culture and sensitivity data, de-escalation and targeted antibiotic therapy should be initiated. However, with the rise in DFIs caused by MRSA, empiric coverage for MRSA needs to considered for both limb-threatening and non-limb-threatening infections, since they both typically contain *S. aureus* isolates.

A recent consensus statement from an expert panel has recommended following the IDSA classification and choosing empiric therapy based on the type of infection: "mild" or "moderate and severe" (16). The algorithm is illustrated in Figure 1. This is a guide for *empiric* therapy of DFIs while awaiting the result of a properly taken culture and sensitivity. In mild infections, which are predominately gram-positive, the outpatient empiric therapy should be based on risk factors for MRSA. If there are no risk factors, one can be treated with a penicillin derivative, a cephalosporin, or clindamycin. If risk factors for MRSA are present, one should

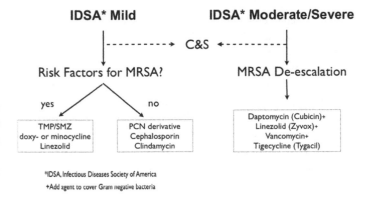

FIGURE 1 Algorithm for the initial empiric treatment of DFIs.

use oral linezolid, minocycline/doxycycline, or trimethoprim/sulfa. The latter two drugs are useful especially if community-acquired MRSA is suspected. Clindamycin is another choice, but it is often avoided as an empiric agent in patients with MRSA risk factors since there is inducible resistance.

In moderate and severe infections, which are typically polymicrobial, the patients are usually hospitalized. Empiric therapy needs to be broad spectrum, and MRSA de-escalation should be initiated, regardless of risk factors (66). Many times, this requires combination drug therapy to achieve this goal, such as intravenous linezolid plus a gram-negative agent, vancomycin plus a gram-negative agent and "double cover" MSSA, or tigecycline monotherapy.

ANTIMICROBIALS FOR MRSA DFIS

Vancomycin, daptomycin, linezolid, tigecycline, and quinupristin-dalfopristin have all been studied for skin and soft tissue infections. Vancomycin has been the historical drug of choice for MRSA DFIs, but with emerging vancomycin-resistant *S. aureus* (VRSA) and *Enterococcus* (VRE) and the renal side effect caused by this drug in an already renally impaired population, its use is being questioned frequently. Chronic ulcers and vancomycin use place one at risk for developing VRSA (67). Although vancomycin is commonly used for diabetic foot osteomylelitis with MRSA, one study evaluating vancomycin for vertebral OM reported that vancomycin alone was not sufficient for resolution (68). Furthermore, there is a high failure rate in MRSA bactremia when vancomycin is used where the MIC is greater than 1.5 (69).

Daptomycin is a lipopeptide antibiotic active against VRE, MRSA, glycopeptideintermediate–susceptible *S. aureus*, and coagulase-negative staphylococci (70). It is FDA approved for use in complicated skin and skin-structure infections (cSSSI) (34). Daptomycin has been studied in infected DFUs and found to be equivalent to vancomycin or a semi-synthetic penicillin (71). Some staphylococcal resistance to daptomycin has recently been reported (72). An in vitro OM model measuring the leeching of antibiotic for vancomycin and daptomycin revealed that both drugs were similar in concentration released (73).

Quinupristin/dalfopristin is a parenteral streptogramin antimicrobial agent with activity against a broad range of gram-positive bacteria including MRSA, VRE, streptococci, *Clostridium perfringens*, and *Peptostreptococcus* spp. (74). It is approved for severe or life-threatening infections associated with VRE. Quinupristin/dalfopristin has not been evaluated for use in DFIs.

Tigecycline is a glycylcycline antibiotic related to the tetracycline group of drugs. It is broad spectrum with activity against MRSA, VRE and multiple gram-negative bacteria, excluding *Pseudomonas* spp. (75). It has been shown to be equivalent to vancomycin plus aztreonam in cSSSI (76). In experimental OM with a rabbit model, tigeclycline plus rifampin showed 100% clearance of OM in four weeks, compared with vancomycin plus rifampin at 90%, and only 26% in the untreated controls (77).

Linezolid, an oxazolidinone, is broadly active against gram-positive bacteria including MRSA and VRE and is FDA approved for cSSTI (78). Linezolid is the only antibiotic with activity against MRSA to have an FDA indication for DFIs. Unlike the other anti-MRSA drugs, linezolid is available in parenteral and oral forms with the oral formation having 100% bioavailability (79). Specifically evaluating lower extremity cSSTI caused by MRSA, Sharp et al. found a greater cure rate and an average of three-day shorter length of stay for linezolid versus vancomycin. Vancomycin was associated with more treatment failures and major amputations (80). In OM, linezolid plus surgical resection and reconstruction was associated with a 90% success rate in 40 patients (81). Rayner et al. found that linezolid was effective in the treatment of OM with an 82% cure rate; however, only 22 of 89 patients were available for follow-up (82).

CONCLUSION

The burden of MRSA in DFIs is increasing causing more treatment failures, increased length of hospital stays, increased health care costs, and more amputations. MRSA DFIs are associated with greater morbidity and mortality. Empiric treatment MRSA needs to be considered in patients with IDSA mild infections and risk factors and those with moderate or severe infections. DNA-based probes can provide rapid identification of MRSA and, when more widely available, will reduce the need for empiric therapy against MRSA. There is a paucity of literature evaluating the treatment of MRSA infections specifically in DFIs. No sufficient evidence exists regarding the use of any anti-MRSA drug in the setting of OM that forces physicians to choose one based on anecdote or safety/adverse effect profile. Caution must be taken as bacterial resistance to these new drugs may develop, especially when being used in the environment of a chronic skin ulcer with polymicrobial colonization. Identification and classification of DFI, de-escalating culture–directed antimicrobial therapy, and addressing the concomitant conditions that delay wound healing can help to prevent LEA in this high-risk population.

REFERENCES

1. Singh N, Armstrong DG, Lipsky BA. Preventing foot ulcers in patients with diabetes. JAMA 2005; 293(2):217–228.
2. Reiber GE, Boyko EJ, Smith DG. Lower extremity foot ulcers and amputations in diabetes. In: Harris MI, Cowie C, Stern MP, eds. Diabetes in America. 2nd ed. Washington, DC: United Government Printing Office (NIH Publ. 95-1468), 1995.
3. Rogers LC, Lavery LA, Armstrong DG. The right to bear legs—an amendment to healthcare: how preventing amputations can save billions to the US health-care system. J Am Pediatr Med Assoc 2008; 98(2):166–168.
4. Pecoraro RE, Reiber GE, Burgess EM. Pathways to diabetic limb amputation: basis for prevention. Diabetes Care 1990; 13:513–521.
5. Armstrong DG, Lavery LA. Diabetic foot ulcers: prevention, diagnosis and classification. Am Fam Phys 1998; 57:1325–1340.
6. Control CfD. Surveillance summary: non-traumatic amputations. 1999; Available at: http://www.cdc.gov/diabetes/statistics/survl99/chap6/contents.htm. Accessed September 6, 2006.
7. Goldner MG. The fate of the second leg in the diabetic amputee. Diabetes 1960; 9:100–103.
8. Jeffcoate WJ, Chipchase SY, Ince P, et al. Assessing the outcome of the management of diabetic foot ulcers using ulcer-related and person-related measures. Diabetes Care 2006; 29(8):1784–1787.
9. Ramsey SD, Newton K, Blough D, et al. Incidence, outcomes, and cost of foot ulcers in patients with diabetes. Diabetes Care 1999; 22(3):382–387.
10. Lavery LA, Armstrong DG, Wunderlich RP, et al. Risk factors for foot infections in individuals with diabetes. Diabetes Care 2006; 29(6):1288–1293.
11. Karchmer AW. Microbiology and treatment of diabetic foot infections. In: Veves A, Giurini JM, LoGerfo FW, eds. The Diabetic Foot. 2nd ed. Totowa, New Jersey: Humana Press, 2006:255–268.
12. Armstrong DG, Lavery LA, Sariaya M, et al. Leukocytosis is a poor indicator of acute osteomyelitis of the foot in diabetes mellitus. J Foot Ankle Surg 1996; 35(4):280–283.

13. McMahon MM, Bistrian BR. Host defenses and susceptibility to infection in patients with diabetes mellitus. Infect Dis Clin North Am 1995; 9(1): 1–9.

14. O'Meara S, Nelson EA, Golder S, et al. Systematic review of methods to diagnose infection in foot ulcers in diabetes. Diabet Med 2006; 23(4):341–347.

15. Lipsky BA, Berendt AR, Deery HG, et al. Diagnosis and treatment of diabetic foot infections. Clin Infect Dis. 2004; 39(7):885–910.

16. Armstrong DG, Boulton AJM, Joseph WS, et al. A closer look at the prevalence of MRSA and its impact on empiric therapy. Wounds 2008; 8(suppl 12):S5–S10.

17. Lavery LA, Armstrong DG, Murdoch DP, et al. Validation of the Infectious Diseases Society of America's diabetic foot infection classification system. Clin Infect Dis 2007; 44(4):562–565.

18. Caputo GM, Cavanagh PR, Ulbrecht JS, et al. Assessment and management of foot disease in patients with diabetes. N Engl J Med 1994; 331(13): 854–860.

19. Armstrong DG, Lavery LA, Harkless LB. Validation of a diabetic wound classification system. The contribution of depth, infection, and ischemia to risk of amputation [see comments]. Diabetes Care 1998; 21(5):855–859.

20. Oyibo SO, Jude EB, Tarawneh I, et al. A comparison of two diabetic foot ulcer classification systems. Diabetes 2000; 49(suppl 1):A33.

21. Grayson ML, Balaugh K, Levin E, et al. Probing to bone in infected pedal ulcers. A clinical sign of underlying osteomyelitis in diabetic patients. J Am Med Assoc 1995; 273(9):721–723.

22. Shone A, Burnside J, Chipchase S, et al. Probing the validity of the probe-to-bone test in the diagnosis of osteomyelitis of the foot in diabetes. Diabetes Care 2006; 29(4):945.

23. El-Maghraby TA, Moustafa HM, Pauwels EK. Nuclear medicine methods for evaluation of skeletal infection among other diagnostic modalities. Q J Nucl Med Mol Imaging 2006; 50(3):167–192.

24. Lipsky BA. A current approach to diabetic foot infections. Curr Infect Dis Rep 1999; 1(3):253–260.

25. Neil JA, Munro CL. A comparison of two culturing methods for chronic wounds. Ostomy Wound Manage 1997; 43(3):20–22, 24, 26 passim.

26. Wheat LJ, Allen SD, Henry M, et al. Diabetic foot infections. Bacteriologic analysis. Arch Intern Med 1986; 146(10):1935–1940.

27. Slater RA, Lazarovitch T, Boldur I, et al. Swab cultures accurately identify bacterial pathogens in diabetic foot wounds not involving bone. Diabet Med 2004; 21(7):705–709.

28. Pellizzer G, Strazzabosco M, Presi S, et al. Deep tissue biopsy vs. superficial swab culture monitoring in the microbiological assessment of limb-threatening diabetic foot infection. Diabet Med 2001; 18(10):822–827.

29. Calhoun JH, Overgaard KA, Stevens CM, et al. Diabetic foot ulcers and infections: current concepts. Adv Skin Wound Care 2002; 15(1):31–42; quiz 44–35.

30. Williams DT, Hilton JR, Harding KG. Diagnosing foot infection in diabetes. Clin Infect Dis 2004; 39(suppl 2):S83–S86.

31. Lipsky BA. Medical treatment of diabetic foot infections. Clin Infect Dis 2004; 39(suppl 2):S104–S114.

32. Grayson ML, Gibbons GW, Habershaw GM, et al. Use of ampicillin/sulbactam versus imipenem/cilastatin in the treatment of limb-threatening foot infections in diabetic patients. Clin Infect Dis 1994; 18(5):683–693.

33. Scher KS, Steele FJ. The septic foot in patients with diabetes. Surgery 1988; 104:661–666.

34. LaPlante KL, Rybak MJ. Daptomycin—a novel antibiotic against Gram-positive pathogens. Expert Opin Pharmacother 2004; 5(11):2321–2331.

35. Tentolouris N, Petrikkos G, Vallianou N, et al. Prevalence of methicillin-resistant *Staphylococcus aureus* in infected and uninfected diabetic foot ulcers. Clin Microbiol Infect 2006; 12(2):186–189.

36. Dang CN, Prasad YD, Boulton AJ, et al. Methicillin-resistant *Staphylococcus aureus* in the diabetic foot clinic: a worsening problem. Diabet Med 2003; 20(2):159–161.

37. Tentolouris N, Jude EB, Smirnof I, et al. Methicillin-resistant *Staphylococcus aureus*: an increasing problem in a diabetic foot clinic. Diabet Med 1999; 16(9):767–771.

38. Roghmann MC, Siddiqui A, Plaisance K, et al. MRSA colonization and the risk of MRSA bacteraemia in hospitalized patients with chronic ulcers. J Hosp Infect 2001; 47(2):98–103.

39. Warshawsky B, Hussain Z, Gregson DB, et al. Hospital- and community-based surveillance of methicillin-resistant *Staphylococcus aureus*: previous hospitalization is the major risk factor. Infect Control Hosp Epidemiol 2000; 21(11):724–727.

40. Jernigan JA, Pullen AL, Flowers L, et al. Prevalence of and risk factors for colonization with methicillin-resistant *Staphylococcus aureus* at the time of hospital admission. Infect Control Hosp Epidemiol 2003; 24(6):409–414.

41. Furuno JP, Harris AD, Wright MO, et al. Prediction rules to identify patients with methicillin-resistant *Staphylococcus aureus* and vancomycin-resistant enterococci upon hospital admission. Am J Infect Control 2004; 32(8): 436–440.

42. Troillet N, Carmeli Y, Samore MH, et al. Carriage of methicillin-resistant *Staphylococcus aureus* at hospital admission. Infect Control Hosp Epidemiol 1998; 19(3):181–185.

43. Vidhani S, Mathur MD, Mehndiratta PL, et al. Methicillin resistant *Staphylococcus aureus* (MRSA): the associated risk factors. Indian J Pathol Microbiol 2003; 46(4):676–679.

44. Huang SS, Platt R. Risk of methicillin-resistant *Staphylococcus aureus* infection after previous infection or colonization. Clin Infect Dis 2003; 36(3): 281–285.

45. Khatib R, Johnson LB, Fakih MG, et al. Persistence in *Staphylococcus aureus* bacteremia: incidence, characteristics of patients and outcome. Scand J Infect Dis 2006; 38(1):7–14.

46. Talon D, Woronoff-Lemsi MC, Limat S, et al. The impact of resistance to methicillin in *Staphylococcus aureus* bacteremia on mortality. Eur J Intern Med 2002; 13(1):31–36.

47. Tsao SM, Hsu CC, Yin MC. Meticillin-resistant *Staphylococcus aureus* infection in diabetic mice enhanced inflammation and coagulation. J Med Microbiol 2006; 55(pt 4):379–385.

48. Miller LG, Perdreau-Remington F, Rieg G, et al. Necrotizing fasciitis caused by community-associated methicillin-resistant *Staphylococcus aureus* in Los Angeles. N Engl J Med 2005; 352(14):1445–1453.

49. Wong CH, Tan SH, Kurup A, et al. Recurrent necrotizing fasciitis caused by methicillin-resistant *Staphylococcus aureus*. Eur J Clin Microbiol Infect Dis 2004; 23(12):909–911.

50. Grimble SA, Magee TR, Galland RB. Methicillin resistant *Staphylococcus aureus* in patients undergoing major amputation. Eur J Vasc Endovasc Surg 2001; 22(3):215–218.

51. Richards T, Pittathankel AA, Pursell R, et al. MRSA in lower limb amputation and the role of antibiotic prophylaxis. J Cardiovasc Surg (Torino) 2005; 46(1):37–41.

52. Boulton AJ, Meneses P, Ennis WJ. Diabetic foot ulcers: a framework for prevention and care. Wound Repair Regen 1999; 7(1):7–16.

53. Rauwerda JA. Foot debridement: anatomic knowledge is mandatory. Diabetes Metab Res Rev 2000; 16(suppl 1):S23–S26.

54. Sibbald RG, Williamson D, Orsted HL, et al. Preparing the wound bed—debridement, bacterial balance, and moisture balance. Ostomy Wound Manage 2000; 46(11):14–22, 24–18, 30–15; quiz 36–17.

55. Attinger CE, Bulan EJ. Debridement. The key initial first step in wound healing. Foot Ankle Clin 2001; 6(4):627–660.

56. Saxena V, Hwang CW, Huang S, et al. Vacuum-assisted closure: micro-deformations of wounds and cell proliferation. Plast Reconstr Surg 2004; 114(5): 1086–1096; discussion 1097–1088.

57. Armstrong DG, Lavery LA. Negative pressure wound therapy after partial diabetic foot amputation: a multicentre, randomised controlled trial. Lancet 2005; 366(9498):1704–1710.

58. Wu SC, Crews RT, Armstrong DG. The pivotal role of offloading in the management of neuropathic foot ulceration. Curr Diab Rep 2005; 5(6): 423–429.

59. Armstrong DG, Lavery LA, Bushman TR. Peak foot pressures influence healing time of diabetic ulcers treated with total contact casting. J Rehabil Res Dev 1998; 35:1–5.

60. Sinacore DR, Mueller MJ, Diamond JE. Diabetic plantar ulcers treated by total contact casting. Phys Ther 1987; 67:1543–1547.

61. Lavery LA, Vela SA, Lavery DC, et al. Reducing dynamic foot pressures in high-risk diabetic subjects with foot ulcerations. A comparison of treatments. Diabetes Care 1996; 19(8):818–821.

62. Armstrong DG, Lavery LA, Kimbriel HR, et al. Activity patterns of patients with diabetic foot ulceration: patients with active ulceration may not adhere to a standard pressure off-loading regimen. Diabetes Care 2003; 26(9): 2595–2597.

63. Armstrong DG, Short B, Nixon BP, et al. Technique for fabrication of an "instant" total contact cast for treatment of neuropathic diabetic foot ulcers. J Am Podiatr Med Assoc 2002; 92:405–408.

64. Harkless L, Boghossian J, Pollak R, et al. An open-label, randomized study comparing efficacy and safety of intravenous piperacillin/tazobactam and ampicillin/sulbactam for infected diabetic foot ulcers. Surg Infect (Larchmt) 2005; 6(1):27–40.

65. Lipsky BA, Armstrong DG, Citron DM, et al. Ertapenem versus piperacillin/tazobactam for diabetic foot infections (SIDESTEP): prospective, randomised, controlled, double-blinded, multicentre trial. Lancet 2005; 366(9498): 1695–1703.

66. Lipsky BA. Empirical therapy for diabetic foot infections: are there clinical clues to guide antibiotic selection? Clin Microbiol Infect 2007; 12:351–353.

67. Appelbaum PC. The emergence of vancomycin-intermediate and vancomycin-resistant *Staphylococcus aureus*. Clin Microbiol Infect 2006; 12(suppl 1): 16–23.

68. Gelfand MS, Cleveland KO. Vancomycin therapy and the progression of methicillin-resistant *Staphylococcus aureus* vertebral osteomyelitis. South Med J 2004; 97(6):593–597.

69. Lodise TP, Graves J, Evans A, et al. Relationship between vancomycin MIC and failure rate among patients with methicillin-resistant *Staphylococcus aureus* bacteremia treated with vancomycin. Antimicrob Agents Chemother 2008; 52:3315–3320.

70. Tally FP, Zeckel M, Wasilewski MM, et al. Daptomycin: a novel agent for Gram-positive infections. Expert Opin Investig Drugs 1999; 8(8):1223–1238.

71. Lipsky BA, Stoutenburgh U. Daptomycin for treating infected diabetic foot ulcers: evidence from a randomized, controlled trial comparing daptomycin with vancomycin or semi-synthetic penicillins for complicated skin and skin-structure infections. J Antimicrob Chemother 2005; 55(2):240–245.

72. Jevitt LA, Thorne GM, Traczewski MM, et al. Multicenter evaluation of the etest and disk diffusion methods for differentiating daptomycin-susceptible from non-daptomycin-susceptible *Staphylococcus aureus* isolates. J Clin Microbiol 2006; 44(9):3098–3104.

73. Rouse MS, Piper KE, Jacobson M, et al. Daptomycin treatment of *Staphylococcus aureus* experimental chronic osteomyelitis. J Antimicrob Chemother 2006; 57(2):301–305.

74. Lamb HM, Figgitt DP, Faulds D. Quinupristin/dalfopristin: a review of its use in the management of serious gram-positive infections. Drugs 1999; 58(6): 1061–1097.

75. Livermore DM. Tigecycline: what is it, and where should it be used? J Antimicrob Chemother 2005; 56(4):611–614.

76. Ellis-Grosse EJ, Babinchak T, Dartois N, et al. The efficacy and safety of tigecycline in the treatment of skin and skin-structure infections: results of 2 double-blind phase 3 comparison studies with vancomycin-aztreonam. Clin Infect Dis 2005; 41(suppl 5):S341–S353.

77. Yin LY, Lazzarini L, Li F, et al. Comparative evaluation of tigecycline and vancomycin, with and without rifampicin, in the treatment of methicillin-resistant *Staphylococcus aureus* experimental osteomyelitis in a rabbit model. J Antimicrob Chemother 2005; 55(6):995–1002.

78. Peppard WJ, Weigelt JA. Role of linezolid in the treatment of complicated skin and soft tissue infections. Expert Rev Anti Infect Ther 2006; 4(3):357–366.
79. Plosker GL, Figgitt DP. Linezolid: a pharmacoeconomic review of its use in serious Gram-positive infections. Pharmacoeconomics 2005; 23(9):945–964.
80. Sharpe JN, Shively EH, Polk HC Jr. Clinical and economic outcomes of oral linezolid versus intravenous vancomycin in the treatment of MRSA-complicated, lower-extremity skin and soft-tissue infections caused by methicillin-resistant *Staphylococcus aureus*. Am J Surg 2005; 189(4):425–428.
81. Broder KW, Moise PA, Schultz RO, et al. Clinical experience with linezolid in conjunction with wound coverage techniques for skin and soft-tissue infections and postoperative osteomyelitis. Ann Plast Surg 2004; 52(4):385–390.
82. Rayner CR, Baddour LM, Birmingham MC, et al. Linezolid in the treatment of osteomyelitis: results of compassionate use experience. Infection 2004; 32(1): 8–14.

Methicillin-Resistant *Staphylococcus aureus* Pneumonia

7

Anna P. Lam and Richard G. Wunderink
Division of Pulmonary and Critical Care Medicine, Northwestern University
Feinberg School of Medicine, Chicago, Illinois U.S.A.

INTRODUCTION

Infections because of multidrug-resistant (MDR) organisms are a burgeoning problem in the treatment of increasingly complex medical patients. Respiratory infections caused by methicillin-resistant *Staphylococcus aureus* (MRSA) are especially challenging. Whether acquired from the community or nosocomially, these highly adaptable bacteria possess distinctive genes for antibiotic resistance and toxins that present significant obstacles to effective care.

The high mortality rate attributed to ventilator-associated pneumonia (VAP) is well documented since the early days of mechanical ventilation. The emergence of MDR pathogens makes this disease even more difficult to treat. Even in young immunocompetent adults, the combination of MRSA and pneumonia, regardless of whether ventilator associated or community acquired, results in one of the most lethal infections. Pneumonia because of MRSA differs from infections with other MDR pathogens and poses unique challenges to successful treatment and prevention.

EPIDEMIOLOGY

Community-Acquired MRSA Pneumonia

Since the first description in a series of intravenous drug users at Henry Ford Hospital in Detroit (1), reports of methicillin resistance in *S. aureus* isolates outside of health care facilities have been on the rise. Unlike nosocomial MRSA, community-acquired MRSA (CA-MRSA) is typically not MDR. However, the strains now circulating in the United States and around the world possess leukocidin, a toxin first described by Panton and Valentine in 1932 (2). Panton-Valentine leukocidin (PVL) was rare, seen in <2% of all strains (3), but consistently more likely to be found in the community than in hospital-acquired strains (4,5). These PVL-positive isolates carry the type IV SCC*mec* element characteristic of CA-MRSA, indicating that these isolates did not emerge from health care–associated pathogens (6,7). The genetic background of CA-MRSA isolates from various continents differs, suggesting simultaneous coevolution rather than dissemination of a single clone (7). However, strains from different areas of the world have different expression of other toxins while all being positive for PVL and type IV SCC*mec* (7).

Interest in PVL has been stimulated by the emergence of CA-MRSA strains carrying this toxin in necrotizing community-acquired pneumonia (CAP) and skin infections (4,8,9). CA-MRSA infections are found in significantly younger patients and are more likely to involve skin and soft tissue than respiratory tract, compared to health care–associated MRSA infections (5). Outbreaks of MRSA-associated skin and soft tissue infections from the community are common across the country (10–15) although at present, only 5% of CA-MRSA isolates are found in invasive infections (13). However, CAP because of MRSA possessing PVL is increasingly reported, often associated with an antecedent influenza-like illness. A very high mortality, up to 37%, is reported despite this condition infecting predominantly young, otherwise healthy patients (6,8,16). Thus, early recognition and appropriate antibiotic therapy are vital for treating CA-MRSA pneumonia.

Health Care–Acquired MRSA Pneumonia

S. aureus, both methicillin-sensitive *S. aureus* (MSSA) and MRSA, is the most frequently isolated pathogen in the ICU (17). Patients with *S. aureus* infections had, on average, three times the length of stay and total charges and five times the risk of inpatient death as patients without *S. aureus* infections (18).

VAP is unfortunately not an uncommon complication for the ICU patient, with incidence rates from 1 to >20 cases per 1000 ventilator days (19). After five days, VAP is more likely to be caused by MDR pathogens, such as MRSA, and is associated with increased mortality rates (17,19–23). The incidence of MRSA as a cause of VAP is 12% to 15% overall, but increases to approximately 30% in patients with prolonged mechanical ventilation and prior antibiotic therapy (24). The incidence does vary from country to country, hospital to hospital (25,26), and even from ICU to ICU (27). Given the frequency of MRSA as a cause of VAP, the initial treatment for VAP in most ICUs should include empiric vancomycin or linezolid (24,28,29).

Attributable mortality of nosocomial pneumonia in intubated and ventilated patients may be 27% with a risk ratio for death of 2.0 (21) although this is driven principally by mortality from nonfermenting gram-negative bacilli. Likely, the attributable mortality for MRSA may be closer to 15% to 20% (30–32). Mortality and attributable costs are consistently higher with MRSA VAP compared to MSSA (33–36).

Health Care–Associated Pneumonia

Health care–associated pneumonia (HCAP) has been recognized as a CAP in patients who carry risk factors for MDR pathogens. The empirical antibiotic regimens recommended for HCAP therefore are more like those for hospital-acquired pneumonia (HAP) than CAP (29). Culture-based studies of HCAP suggest that the incidence of MRSA in HCAP exceeds that of HAP and VAP (37,38).

MRSA pneumonia, whether community acquired or nosocomial, is a significant health care burden, requiring effective prevention and treatment strategies in order to decrease the associated mortality and morbidity. Despite limited therapeutic options, lively debate and controversy in this field abounds. The current state of therapeutic options and preventive measures, including identification of known risk factors, will be reviewed.

RISK FACTORS FOR DEVELOPMENT OF MRSA PNEUMONIA

Nasal Carriage of *Staphylococcus aureus*

S. aureus is a human commensal organism that commonly colonizes the anterior nares. Up to 80% of the population are constant or intermittent carriers (39), including health care workers as well as patients. The bacteria can be carried in the nares for more than one year, with a half-life of colonization of MRSA around 40 months (40). Nasal carriage, rather than skin colonization, is an important risk factor for invasive disease (39,41,42). Conversely, absence of nasal colonization is associated with less than 5% risk of subsequent MRSA pneumonia (43). The association with nasal carriage may not be as strong for CA-MRSA infections (43), with the skin being another potential site of colonization (44). This high frequency of colonization of both patients and their caregivers is unique from other MDR pathogens. In addition, nasal colonization requires prevention strategies different from gastrointestinal colonization or environmental contamination (45).

Prior Antibiotic Therapy

The major predisposing factor for CA-MRSA, rather than MSSA, is likely the same as for nosocomial MRSA—prior antibiotic therapy (9,25,46). Antibiotics offer a selective advantage for the small number of antibiotic-resistant mutants already present in large inoculums. Early-onset MSSA VAP was found in only 14.6% of patients who did not receive prior antibiotics; none of these patients developed MRSA VAP (24). Even in patients with prolonged ($\geq$7 days) mechanical ventilation, the rate of MSSA VAP was 21.9% while MRSA VAP was only 3.1% if patients had not received any prior antibiotics. In contrast, in those patients with antibiotic exposure in the previous 15 days, 4.6% and 19.7% of patients developed MSSA VAP and MRSA VAP, respectively (24). The type of antibiotic exposure may also play a role. Data from 17 U.S. hospitals showed a significant association between total inpatient fluoroquinolone use and percentage of MRSA isolated (47). Similar associations are seen with macrolide and third-generation cephalosporin use (48).

Nursing home patients are more likely to have MRSA VAP or HCAP. Once again, the major risk factor is prior antibiotic therapy, selecting for MDR pathogens in general (49). The increased percentage of MRSA in nursing homes correlates with increased quinolone but decreased trimethoprim-sulfamethoxazole use (50). Nasal carriage rates were also associated with prior antibiotic use in elderly residents of a nursing home (51).

Prolonged Mechanical Ventilation

The length of mechanical ventilation is a risk factor for development of MRSA VAP. During a five-year outbreak of MRSA in a university teaching hospital, MRSA VAP only occurred after $\geq$3 ventilator days (52). Other studies concur that while MRSA can cause early-onset VAP, the incidence of MRSA in late-onset ($\geq$6 days) pneumonia is increased (20,33). Patients ventilated for a prolonged period ($\geq$6 days) have a twofold relative risk for developing MRSA VAP (33).

Poor Infection Control

The emergence of antibiotic-resistant pathogens, such as MRSA, is linked to breaches in infection control measures, such as noncompliance with handwashing and isolation precaution recommendations (17,53). Poor hygiene and infection control in military recruits and inmates contribute to MRSA outbreaks (10,54). The presence of more than two patients having nasal MRSA colonization in the same ICU at the same time was associated with increased MRSA infections (55). Aggressive screening, contact precautions, and use of alcohol handrub solutions, even in ICUs with high prevalence of MRSA at admission, reduced the spread to exposed patients (56).

Head Trauma/Coma

Patients with head injury and critically ill comatose patients are at increased risk for developing VAP (57,58). This event seems to occur early (<7 days) during the course of mechanical ventilation (57,59,60). The most frequently isolated organism from these early onset pneumonias was *S. aureus* (58–60). Colonization of the nares, pharynx, and trachea with *S. aureus* was further associated with early onset VAP in patients with head injuries (61–63).

Prior Viral Infection

The incidence of *S. aureus* CAP is increased during influenza epidemics in general. The new PVL-containing strains of CA-MRSA were highly associated with a preceding viral illness when presenting as pneumonia (6,8,16). More recent data has suggested that CA-MRSA is not just a postinfluenza infection but lack of concomitant influenza is associated with lower mortality (64). Experimental rhinovirus infection has also been shown to increase the shedding of *S. aureus* (65).

TREATMENT OPTIONS

Antimicrobial agents active against MRSA are limited. In the glycopeptide family, vancomycin is the best known in the United States. Teicoplanin is similar to vancomycin but unavailable in the United States.

Teicoplanin has a longer half-life than vancomycin and can be given intramuscularly (66). Although these two glycopeptides have never undergone a randomized controlled trial to demonstrate their efficacy in MRSA pneumonia, both have become the de facto standards since, until recently, no other viable alternatives existed.

Vancomycin/Teicoplanin

The efficacy of glycopeptide treatment, in general, and vancomycin, in particular, for lower respiratory tract infections (LRTI) remains controversial. Vancomycin intrinsically is less effective against staphylococci than β-lactam antibiotics (66–68). Infection-associated mortality among patients with MSSA pneumonia was significantly higher for those treated with vancomycin than cloxacillin (47% vs. 0%, respectively) (34). Among the patients with *S. aureus* LRTI, vancomycin clinical success was only 54%, even though 58% had MRSA, while all antibacterials other than vancomycin had a 71% clinical success rate, including a 100% clinical success rate in patients with MSSA pneumonia treated with oxacillin (69).

The clinical cure rates specifically for vancomycin treatment of MRSA HAP are seen in the Figure 1 (46,70–72). No study has documented a clinical success rate greater than 65%, and significantly lower rates are found when only VAP is included. Inappropriate initial empiric therapy does not appear to be the reason for failure since no difference in mortality was found even if vancomycin therapy was delayed up to 48 hours from the initial diagnosis (46).

Vancomycin is ineffective at clearing bacteria from the lower respiratory tract. Repeat quantitative cultures demonstrated that only 15% of patients with MRSA VAP treated with vancomycin had decreased colony counts below diagnostic thresholds (73). This finding contrasts with 85% sterile repeat cultures when VAP was due to other microorganisms. Failure to clear the bacteria within the first several days of treatment, not surprisingly, was associated with increased 28-day mortality (73). This

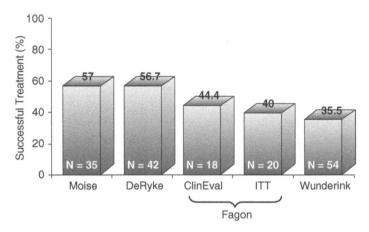

FIGURE 1 Clinical success of vancomycin treatment of methicillin-resistant *Staphylococcus aureus* ventilator-associated pneumonia.

retrospective analysis was recently confirmed by a prospective randomized trial comparing linezolid to vancomycin (74). While bacterial clearance [as documented by a repeat bronchoalveolar lavage (BAL) after 3 to 4 days of therapy] was not significantly different, 50% of patients who failed to decrease BAL colony counts below 100 CFU/mL with vancomycin died. Failure to clear with linezolid was not associated with either clinical failure or mortality.

One potential explanation for the poor clinical outcomes with vancomycin treatment of *S. aureus* pneumonia is the degree of penetration into lung tissue. Homogenized lung tissue from patients undergoing lung resection had low vancomycin levels compared to serum (lung to serum ratio 0.21) (75). By 3 hours post infusion, a substantial portion of patients had lung vancomycin levels below the minimal inhibitory concentration (MIC), and at 12 hours post infusion, almost half had no detectable level. In intubated patients with suspected pneumonia, the

BAL vancomycin concentration was only 25% of serum (76). When albumin concentration in BAL was used as a marker of inflammation, higher levels (>3.4 mg/mL) were associated with slightly higher vancomycin levels but still at only a fraction of the serum level. More than half of MRSA VAP patients given vancomycin 30 mg/kg, dosed every six hours, had BAL vancomycin levels that were undetectable after four doses; in the remaining patients, mean BAL vancomycin concentration was 2.0 μg/mL with corresponding serum levels of 22.2 μg/mL and trough levels above 20 μg/mL (77).

One response to limited lung levels of vancomycin is to increase dosing, since the overwhelming majority of studies showing poor outcome with vancomycin have used doses of 2 g/day or less. Higher doses of vancomycin, as measured by the area under the concentration curve, did appear to correlate with the outcome (78). However, clinical success is also dependent on the MIC of the isolate. If the vancomycin MIC is 1 to 2 μg/mL, the success rate is less than 10% (79). High failure rates with vancomycin MICs of 2 μg/mL are also documented for other serious MRSA infections (80). For bacteremia, mortality in patients receiving vancomycin for MRSA with an MIC of 2 μg/mL had a mortality rate equivalent to patients who did not receive initial MRSA coverage. The consistency of the relationship between MIC and clinical failure suggests that the threshold for vancomycin "sensitivity" may be too high.

An alternative is continuous infusion of vancomycin. A pilot study did not show significant improvement in outcome (81), while multivariate analysis of outcome from MRSA VAP suggests some benefit (32). Higher dosing or continuous infusion is more likely to be associated with renal toxicity. No prospective or randomized trial has demonstrated that higher doses than the standard FDA-approved dose of vancomycin will result in better outcome for MRSA VAP. The presence of an *agr* II polymorphism in MRSA isolates may result in failure no matter what the dose of vancomycin is (82). No evidence suggests that teicoplanin results in any better outcome (83).

An alternative strategy is to look for synergism. Concomitant rifampin or aminoglycosides have not been studied in pneumonia cases but anecdotally have not improved outcome. Compassionate use of quinupristin/dalfopristin plus vancomycin eradicated infection in five patients who had failed glycopeptide monotherapy for non-vancomycin-intermediate *S. aureus* (VISA) nonpneumonic MRSA infection (84).

The response to vancomycin, at least with the standard dose of 2 g/day, is clearly not ideal. Alternative agents have therefore been studied.

Linezolid

Linezolid is an oxazolidone, whose mechanism of action interferes with the assembly of the initiation complex for protein translation by binding to the ribosomal 50S subunit (66,83,85,86). Linezolid was compared to vancomycin in two double-blinded, randomized controlled trials for treatment of suspected gram-positive nosocomial pneumonia (31,72). The first study of 402 patients demonstrated equivalent clinical outcomes between the linezolid and vancomycin groups, with clinical cure rates of 66% and 68%, respectively (72). Unfortunately, only a limited number of patients with MRSA pneumonia were enrolled (only nine patients in the vancomycin group). However, the FDA released linezolid for treatment of suspected gram-positive nosocomial pneumonia on the basis of this trial.

The second larger trial enrolled an additional 623 patients with nosocomial pneumonia, with a larger number of MRSA cases (31). Although no significant clinical outcome difference was demonstrated in the entire population, the subgroup of MRSA pneumonia patients had 20% better clinical cure rates with linezolid than those treated with vancomycin. The survival rate was also greater in the subset of patients with APACHE-II scores of 16 to 19 treated with linezolid.

Since the real indication for treatment of pneumonia with either of these antibiotics is MRSA pneumonia, data from the subset of patients with MRSA pneumonia from both studies was combined for analysis

(87). Significantly higher clinical cure rates were found with linezolid than vancomycin (59% vs. 35%). Logistic regression analysis confirmed linezolid therapy as a significant predictor of clinical cure in MRSA nosocomial pneumonia, along with single-lobe pneumonia, absence of oncologic and renal comorbidities, and absence of VAP. Logistic regression analysis specifically of MRSA VAP confirmed that linezolid treatment remained a significant predictor of clinical cure. The rates for clinical cure were 62% for linezolid versus 21% for vancomycin ($p = 0.001$) (88). Outcome in VAP confirmed by invasive procedures or blood cultures followed the same pattern as the overall group. Most significant was documentation of a significant survival benefit of linezolid over vancomycin (85% vs. 67%) (87). A subsequent small but head-to-head randomized controlled trial of microbiologic response confirmed the differences between linezolid and vancomycin for clinical response and mortality (74).

Several reasons for the superior response to linezolid are possible. Linezolid has a high volume of distribution and penetrates well into tissue (89). Steady-state levels in uninfected patients showed mean linezolid levels in BAL and alveolar macrophages were 25.09 and 8.10 mg/L, respectively (90). In another cohort of healthy volunteers, steady-state BAL levels were four times greater than serum levels at all time points after dosing (91). The concentration of linezolid in epithelial lining fluid remained above the MIC for *S. aureus* 100% of the time during the 12-hour dosing interval and out to 24 hours after the last dose. Data from patients with suspected VAP found BAL/serum ratios closer to one, although a nonstandardized nonbronchoscopic BAL technique was used (92).

For CA-MRSA pneumonia, no randomized clinical trials specifically address the antibiotic choice in this group. Linezolid, because of its mechanism of action, interferes with toxin production (93,94), while vancomycin and teicoplanin do not (95). This factor may be critical when necrotizing pneumonia is present.

None of the main adverse side effects of linezolid, which include neuropathy (optic and peripheral), myelosuppression, and potential monoamine oxidase inhibition, were seen in the clinical trial for pneumonia. The easiest adverse response to detect, thrombocytopenia, was comparable to that of vancomycin (96). Most adverse effects require a longer exposure than the seven- to eight-day treatment for VAP.

Other Therapies

The recent CA-MRSA outbreaks have stimulated interest in older drugs with in vitro susceptibility, such as minocycline and trimethoprim-sulfamethoxazole (85). Levaquin and moxifloxacin appear to be effective against CA-MRSA skin infections. None of these agents has been studied in MRSA pneumonia, especially nosocomial. Concern about rapid development of resistance with fluoroquinolones exists (97). Conversely, necrotic tissue may allow bypass of the folate metabolism block induced by trimethoprim-sulfamethoxazole and render it less effective (98). Addition of clindamycin to vancomycin for CA-MRSA may be effective in suppressing toxin production (94), although monotherapy is likely to lead to emergence of resistance.

Quinupristin/dalfopristin was compared to vancomycin in a prospective, randomized, multicenter trial in patients with gram-positive nosocomial pneumonia (71). While overall clinical success rates were equivalent, outcome in the subpopulation with MRSA was even worse than with vancomycin.

Daptomycin, a promising new cyclic lipopeptide antibiotic, was found to be inferior to a cephalosporin for CAP (99). Most likely this results from inactivation of daptomycin by pulmonary surfactant (100). Tigecycline, a glycylcycline antibiotic (analog of tetracycline), has already been released for complicated skin and intra-abdominal infections (85,101) but data to support its use in MRSA pneumonia are lacking.

A variety of new antibiotics with activity against MRSA are being evaluated. Telavancin, a new glycopeptide (102,103), may have superior outcomes to vancomycin in pneumonia but has not been compared to linezolid. Cephalosporins (ceftaroline and ceftobiprole) with activity against MRSA are now in clinical trials.

PREVENTION STRATEGIES

General

General VAP prevention strategies apply to prevention of MRSA VAP as well. Avoidance of intubation with selective use of noninvasive ventilation, sedation holidays and protocolized weaning strategies, elevating the head of the bed, and appropriate infection control strategies are all important (29). Use of accurate diagnostic strategies to avoid excessive or unneeded antibiotics can also decrease the incidence of MRSA pneumonia, at least as measured by a decrease in the overall use of glycopeptides (104).

Prevention of CA-MRSA outbreaks is based on education of health care providers and adherence to basic infection control principles. Limited data from correctional facilities, military recruits, and competitive sports participants suggest that basic personal and environmental hygiene interventions are effective in controlling outbreaks (10,12,54).

Decreasing *Staphylococcus aureus* Colonization

The only aspect of prevention of VAP specific to MRSA VAP is addressing nasal and subsequent oropharyngeal colonization with *S. aureus*. Mupirocin is a product of *Pseudomonas fluorescens* and inhibits isoleucyl-tRNA synthetase (66). Only available topically, mupirocin has been recommended for clearance of nasal MRSA carriage during outbreaks. In a nonepidemic setting, eradication of MRSA nasal carriage with mupirocin ranged from 44% to 100%, but extranasal eradication was poor (105,106). Recurrence of nasal colonization after decontamination was high and decontamination did not appear to decrease the incidence of subsequent MRSA infection (45).

Selective decontamination of the digestive tract (SDD) decreases mortality and the risk of infection, pneumonia as well as bloodstream, in some studies (107,108). While SDD seems to decrease the rates of MDR gram-negative bacteria, the data regarding the impact of SDD on the emergence of MRSA are conflicting (109–112). Topical vancomycin gel in the oropharynx alone significantly reduced the incidence of MRSA VAP without concomitant increase in the incidence of vancomycin-resistant organisms (113–115). More aggressive approaches focused on decreasing MRSA colonization (116), but the long-term effects of antibiotic prophylaxis remain unclear.

CONCLUSIONS

All categories of pneumonia, HAP, VAP, HCAP, and CAP, because of MRSA pose significant treatment problems. These fascinating bacteria have evolved many mechanisms of virulence and resistance to conventional antibiotics. Current data suggests that linezolid is a superior treatment choice for MRSA VAP in terms of pulmonary penetration and clinical efficacy. No study specifically addresses treatment of CA-MRSA CAP, so treatment is based on extrapolation from the HAP data, with consideration of effects on toxin production. New therapies are emerging, but since further antimicrobial resistance to vancomycin and linezolid is expected, further research is needed to establish the best approach to prevent and eradicate MRSA. In the interim, judicious use of appropriate antibiotics is crucial not only in the effective treatment of MDR pneumonias but also in the prevention of future complications.

REFERENCES

1. Saravolatz LD, Markowitz N, Arking L, et al. Methicillin-resistant *Staphylococcus aureus*. Epidemiologic observations during a community-acquired outbreak. Ann Intern Med 1982; 96(1):11–16.

2. Panton PN, Valentine, FCO. Staphylococcal toxin. Lancet 1932; 1:506–508.

3. Lindsay JA, Holden MT. *Staphylococcus aureus*: superbug, super genome? Trends Microbiol 2004; 12(8):378–385.

4. Lina G, Piemont Y, Godail-Gamot F, et al. Involvement of Panton-Valentine leukocidin-producing *Staphylococcus aureus* in primary skin infections and pneumonia. Clin Infect Dis 1999; 29(5):1128–1132.

5. Naimi TS, LeDell KH, Como-Sabetti K, et al. Comparison of community- and health care-associated methicillin-resistant *Staphylococcus aureus* infection. JAMA 2003; 290(22):2976–2984.

6. Francis JS, Doherty MC, Lopatin U, et al. Severe community-onset pneumonia in healthy adults caused by methicillin-resistant *Staphylococcus aureus* carrying the Panton-Valentine leukocidin genes. Clin Infect Dis 2005; 40(1):100–107.

7. Vandenesch F, Naimi T, Enright MC, et al. Community-acquired methicillin-resistant *Staphylococcus aureus* carrying Panton-Valentine leukocidin genes: worldwide emergence. Emerg Infect Dis 2003; 9(8):978–984.

8. Gillet Y, Issartel B, Vanhems P, et al. Association between *Staphylococcus aureus* strains carrying gene for Panton-Valentine leukocidin and highly lethal necrotising pneumonia in young immunocompetent patients. Lancet 2002; 359(9308):753–759.

9. Ellis MW, Hospenthal DR, Dooley DP, et al. Natural history of community-acquired methicillin-resistant *Staphylococcus aureus* colonization and infection in soldiers. Clin Infect Dis 2004; 39(7):971–979.

10. Centers for Disease Control and Prevention (CDC). Methicillin-resistant *Staphylococcus aureus* infections in correctional facilities—Georgia, California, and Texas, 2001–2003. MMWR Morb Mortal Wkly Rep 2003; 52(41):992–996.

11. Schaaf BM, Boehmke F, Esnaashari H, et al. Pneumococcal septic shock is associated with the interleukin-10-1082 gene promoter polymorphism. Am J Respir Crit Care Med 2003; 168(4):476–480.

12. Gentile DA, Doyle WJ, Zeevi A, et al. Cytokine gene polymorphisms moderate illness severity in infants with respiratory syncytial virus infection. Hum Immunol 2003; 64(3):338–344.

13. Kaplan SL, Hulten KG, Gonzalez BE, et al. Three-year surveillance of community-acquired *Staphylococcus aureus* infections in children. Clin Infect Dis 2005; 40(12):1785–1791.
14. Frazee BW, Lynn J, Charlebois ED, et al. High prevalence of methicillin-resistant *Staphylococcus aureus* in emergency department skin and soft tissue infections. Ann Emerg Med 2005; 45(3):311–320.
15. Young DM, Harris HW, Charlebois ED, et al. An epidemic of methicillin-resistant *Staphylococcus aureus* soft tissue infections among medically underserved patients. Arch Surg 2004; 139(9):947–951; discussion 51–53.
16. Hageman JC, Uyeki TM, Francis JS, et al. Severe community-acquired pneumonia due to *Staphylococcus aureus*, 2003–04 influenza season. Emerg Infect Dis 2006; 12(6):894–899.
17. McGahee W, Lowy FD. Staphylococcal infections in the intensive care unit. Semin Respir Infect 2000; 15(4):308–313.
18. Noskin GA, Rubin RJ, Schentag JJ, et al. The burden of *Staphylococcus aureus* infections on hospitals in the United States: an analysis of the 2000 and 2001 Nationwide Inpatient Sample Database. Arch Intern Med 2005; 165(15):1756–1761.
19. Hubmayr RD, Burchardi H, Elliot M, et al. Statement of the 4th International Consensus Conference in Critical Care on ICU-Acquired Pneumonia—Chicago, Illinois, May 2002. Intensive Care Med 2002; 28(11):1521–1536.
20. Fridkin SK. Increasing prevalence of antimicrobial resistance in intensive care units. Crit Care Med 2001; 29(suppl 4):N64–N68.
21. Fagon JY, Chastre J, Hance AJ, et al. Nosocomial pneumonia in ventilated patients: a cohort study evaluating attributable mortality and hospital stay. Am J Med 1993; 94(3):281–288.
22. Heyland DK, Cook DJ, Griffith L, et al. The attributable morbidity and mortality of ventilator-associated pneumonia in the critically ill patient. The Canadian Critical Trials Group. Am J Respir Crit Care Med 1999; 159(4 pt 1): 1249–1256.
23. Torres A, Carlet J. Ventilator-associated pneumonia. European Task Force on ventilator-associated pneumonia. Eur Respir J 2001; 17(5):1034–1045.
24. Trouillet JL, Chastre J, Vuagnat A, et al. Ventilator-associated pneumonia caused by potentially drug-resistant bacteria. Am J Respir Crit Care Med 1998; 157(2):531–539.
25. Rello J, Sa-Borges M, Correa H, et al. Variations in etiology of ventilator-associated pneumonia across four treatment sites: implications for antimicrobial prescribing practices. Am J Respir Crit Care Med 1999; 160(2):608–613.

26. Babcock HM, Zack JE, Garrison T, et al. Ventilator-associated pneumonia in a multi-hospital system: differences in microbiology by location. Infect Control Hosp Epidemiol 2003; 24(11):853–858.
27. Namias N, Samiian L, Nino D, et al. Incidence and susceptibility of pathogenic bacteria vary between intensive care units within a single hospital: implications for empiric antibiotic strategies. J Trauma 2000; 49(4): 638–645; discussion 45–46.
28. Ibrahim EH, Ward S, Sherman G, et al. Experience with a clinical guideline for the treatment of ventilator-associated pneumonia. Crit Care Med 2001; 29(6):1109–1115.
29. American Thoracic Society; Infectious Diseases Society of America. Guidelines for the management of adults with hospital-acquired, ventilator-associated, and healthcare-associated pneumonia. Am J Respir Crit Care Med 2005; 171(4):388–416.
30. Fagon JY, Chastre J, Domart Y, et al. Nosocomial pneumonia in patients receiving continuous mechanical ventilation. Prospective analysis of 52 episodes with use of a protected specimen brush and quantitative culture techniques. Am Rev Respir Dis 1989; 139(4):877–884.
31. Wunderink RG, Cammarata SK, Oliphant TH, et al. Continuation of a randomized, double-blind, multicenter study of linezolid versus vancomycin in the treatment of patients with nosocomial pneumonia. Clin Ther 2003; 25(3): 980–992.
32. Rello J, Sole-Violan J, Sa-Borges M, et al. Pneumonia caused by oxacillin-resistant *Staphylococcus aureus* treated with glycopeptides. Crit Care Med 2005; 33(9):1983–1987.
33. Rello J, Torres A, Ricart M, et al. Ventilator-associated pneumonia by *Staphylococcus aureus*. Comparison of methicillin-resistant and methicillin-sensitive episodes. Am J Respir Crit Care Med 1994; 150(6 pt 1):1545–1549.
34. Gonzalez C, Rubio M, Romero-Vivas J, et al. Bacteremic pneumonia due to *Staphylococcus aureus*: a comparison of disease caused by methicillin-resistant and methicillin-susceptible organisms. Clin Infect Dis 1999; 29(5): 1171–1177.
35. Cosgrove SE, Sakoulas G, Perencevich EN, et al. Comparison of mortality associated with methicillin-resistant and methicillin-susceptible *Staphylococcus aureus* bacteremia: a meta-analysis. Clin Infect Dis 2003; 36(1):53–59.
36. Shorr AF, Tabak YP, Gupta V, et al. Morbidity and cost burden of methicillin-resistant *Staphylococcus aureus* in early onset ventilator-associated pneumonia. Crit Care 2006; 10(3):R97.

37. Kollef MH, Shorr A, Tabak YP, et al. Epidemiology and outcomes of health-care-associated pneumonia: results from a large US database of culture-positive pneumonia. Chest 2005; 128(6):3854–3862.

38. Micek ST, Kollef KE, Reichley RM, et al. Health care-associated pneumonia and community-acquired pneumonia: a single-center experience. Antimicrob Agents Chemother 2007; 51(10):3568–3573.

39. Foster TJ. The *Staphylococcus aureus* "superbug." J Clin Invest 2004; 114 (12):1693–1696.

40. Sanford MD, Widmer AF, Bale MJ, et al. Efficient detection and long-term persistence of the carriage of methicillin-resistant *Staphylococcus aureus*. Clin Infect Dis 1994; 19(6):1123–1128.

41. Huang SS, Platt R. Risk of methicillin-resistant *Staphylococcus aureus* infection after previous infection or colonization. Clin Infect Dis 2003; 36 (3):281–285.

42. Garrouste-Orgeas M, Timsit JF, Kallel H, et al. Colonization with methicillin-resistant *Staphylococcus aureus* in ICU patients: morbidity, mortality, and glycopeptide use. Infect Control Hosp Epidemiol 2001; 22 (11):687–692.

43. Robicsek A, Suseno M, Beaumont JL, et al. Prediction of methicillin-resistant *Staphylococcus aureus* involvement in disease sites by concomitant nasal sampling. J Clin Microbiol 2008; 46(2):588–592.

44. Hota B, Ellenbogen C, Hayden MK, et al. Community-associated methicillin-resistant *Staphylococcus aureus* skin and soft tissue infections at a public hospital: do public housing and incarceration amplify transmission? Arch Intern Med 2007; 167(10):1026–1033.

45. Robicsek A, Beaumont JL, Thomson RB Jr., Topical therapy for methicillin-resistant *Staphylococcus aureus* colonization: impact on infection risk. Infect Control Hosp Epidemiol 2009; 30(7):623–632.

46. Deryke CA, Lodise TP Jr., Rybak MJ, et al. Epidemiology, treatment, and outcomes of nosocomial bacteremic *Staphylococcus aureus* pneumonia. Chest 2005; 128(3):1414–1422.

47. MacDougall C, Powell JP, Johnson CK, et al. Hospital and community fluoroquinolone use and resistance in *Staphylococcus aureus* and *Escherichia coli* in 17 US hospitals. Clin Infect Dis 2005; 41(4):435–440.

48. Monnet DL, MacKenzie FM, Lopez-Lozano JM, et al. Antimicrobial drug use and methicillin-resistant *Staphylococcus aureus*, Aberdeen, 1996–2000. Emerg Infect Dis 2004; 10(8):1432–1441.

49. El-Solh AA, Pietrantoni C, Bhat A, et al. Microbiology of severe aspiration pneumonia in institutionalized elderly. Am J Respir Crit Care Med 2003; 167(12):1650–1654.

50. Drinka PJ, Gauerke C, Le D. Antimicrobial use and methicillin-resistant *Staphylococcus aureus* in a large nursing home. J Am Med Dir Assoc 2004; 5(4):256–258.

51. Mendelson G, Yearmack Y, Granot E, et al. *Staphylococcus aureus* carrier state among elderly residents of a long-term care facility. J Am Med Dir Assoc 2003; 4(3):125–127.

52. Pujol M, Corbella X, Pena C, et al. Clinical and epidemiological findings in mechanically-ventilated patients with methicillin-resistant *Staphylococcus aureus* pneumonia. Eur J Clin Microbiol Infect Dis 1998; 17(9):622–628.

53. Ho PL. Carriage of methicillin-resistant *Staphylococcus aureus*, ceftazidime-resistant Gram-negative bacilli, and vancomycin-resistant enterococci before and after intensive care unit admission. Crit Care Med 2003; 31(4):1175–1182.

54. Zinderman CE, Conner B, Malakooti MA, et al. Community-acquired methicillin-resistant *Staphylococcus aureus* among military recruits. Emerg Infect Dis 2004; 10(5):941–944.

55. Oztoprak N, Cevik MA, Akinci E, et al. Risk factors for ICU-acquired methicillin-resistant *Staphylococcus aureus* infections. Am J Infect Control 2006; 34(1):1–5.

56. Lucet JC, Paoletti X, Lolom I, et al. Successful long-term program for controlling methicillin-resistant *Staphylococcus aureus* in intensive care units. Intensive Care Med 2005; 31(8):1051–1057.

57. Hsieh AH, Bishop MJ, Kubilis PS, et al. Pneumonia following closed head injury. Am Rev Respir Dis 1992; 146(2):290–294.

58. Rello J, Ausina V, Ricart M, et al. Nosocomial pneumonia in critically ill comatose patients: need for a differential therapeutic approach. Eur Respir J 1992; 5(10):1249–1253.

59. Berrouane Y, Daudenthun I, Riegel B, et al. Early onset pneumonia in neurosurgical intensive care unit patients. J Hosp Infect 1998; 40(4):275–280.

60. Bronchard R, Albaladejo P, Brezac G, et al. Early onset pneumonia: risk factors and consequences in head trauma patients. Anesthesiology 2004; 100(2): 234–239.

61. Campbell W, Hendrix E, Schwalbe R, et al. Head-injured patients who are nasal carriers of *Staphylococcus aureus* are at high risk for *Staphylococcus aureus* pneumonia. Crit Care Med 1999; 27(4):798–801.

62. Ewig S, Torres A, El-Ebiary M, et al. Bacterial colonization patterns in mechanically ventilated patients with traumatic and medical head injury. Incidence, risk factors, and association with ventilator-associated pneumonia. Am J Respir Crit Care Med 1999; 159(1):188–198.

63. Sirvent JM, Torres A, Vidaur L, et al. Tracheal colonisation within 24 h of intubation in patients with head trauma: risk factor for developing early-onset ventilator-associated pneumonia. Intensive Care Med 2000; 26(9): 1369–1372.

64. Kallen AJ, Hageman J, Gorwitz R, et al. Characteristics of *Staphylococcus aureus* community-acquired pneumonia during the 2006–2007 influenza season. Clin Infect Dis 2007; 45(12):1655.

65. Bassetti S, Bischoff WE, Walter M, et al. Dispersal of *Staphylococcus aureus* into the air associated with a rhinovirus infection. Infect Control Hosp Epidemiol 2005; 26(2):196–203.

66. Chambers HF. Methicillin resistance in staphylococci: molecular and biochemical basis and clinical implications. Clin Microbiol Rev 1997; 10(4): 781–791.

67. Lowy FD. *Staphylococcus aureus* infections. N Engl J Med 1998; 339(8): 520–532.

68. Levine DP, Fromm BS, Reddy BR. Slow response to vancomycin or vancomycin plus rifampin in methicillin-resistant *Staphylococcus aureus* endocarditis. Ann Intern Med 1991; 115(9):674–680.

69. Moise-Broder PA, Forrest A, Birmingham MC, et al. Pharmacodynamics of vancomycin and other antimicrobials in patients with *Staphylococcus aureus* lower respiratory tract infections. Clin Pharmacokinet 2004; 43(13): 925–942.

70. Moise PA, Forrest A, Birmingham MC, et al. The efficacy and safety of linezolid as treatment for *Staphylococcus aureus* infections in compassionate use patients who are intolerant of, or who have failed to respond to, vancomycin. J Antimicrob Chemother 2002; 50(6):1017–1026.

71. Fagon J, Patrick H, Haas DW, et al. Treatment of gram-positive nosocomial pneumonia. Prospective randomized comparison of quinupristin/dalfopristin versus vancomycin. Nosocomial Pneumonia Group. Am J Respir Crit Care Med 2000; 161(3 pt 1):753–762.

72. Rubinstein E, Cammarata S, Oliphant T, et al. Linezolid (PNU-100766) versus vancomycin in the treatment of hospitalized patients with nosocomial pneumonia: a randomized, double-blind, multicenter study. Clin Infect Dis 2001; 32(3):402–412.

73. Baughman RP, Kerr MA. Ventilator-associated pneumonia patients who do not reduce bacteria from the lungs have a worse prognosis. J Intensive Care Med 2003; 18(5):269–274.

74. Wunderink RG, Mendelson MH, Somero MS, et al. Early microbiological response to linezolid vs vancomycin in ventilator-associated pneumonia due to methicillin-resistant *Staphylococcus aureus*. Chest 2008; 134(6): 1200–1207.

75. Cruciani M, Gatti G, Lazzarini L, et al. Penetration of vancomycin into human lung tissue. J Antimicrob Chemother 1996; 38(5):865–869.

76. Lamer C, de Beco V, Soler P, et al. Analysis of vancomycin entry into pulmonary lining fluid by bronchoalveolar lavage in critically ill patients. Antimicrob Agents Chemother 1993; 37(2):281–286.

77. Georges H, Leroy O, Alfandari S, et al. Pulmonary disposition of vancomycin in critically ill patients. Eur J Clin Microbiol Infect Dis 1997; 16(5): 385–388.

78. Moise PA, Forrest A, Bhavnani SM, et al. Area under the inhibitory curve and a pneumonia scoring system for predicting outcomes of vancomycin therapy for respiratory infections by *Staphylococcus aureus*. Am J Health Syst Pharm 2000; 57(suppl 2):S4–S9.

79. Sakoulas G, Moise-Broder PA, Schentag J, et al. Relationship of MIC and bactericidal activity to efficacy of vancomycin for treatment of methicillin-resistant *Staphylococcus aureus* bacteremia. J Clin Microbiol 2004; 42(6): 2398–2402.

80. Soriano A, Marco F, Martinez JA, et al. Influence of vancomycin minimum inhibitory concentration on the treatment of methicillin-resistant *Staphylococcus aureus* bacteremia. Clin Infect Dis 2008; 46(2):193–200.

81. Wysocki M, Delatour F, Faurisson F, et al. Continuous versus intermittent infusion of vancomycin in severe staphylococcal infections: prospective multicenter randomized study. Antimicrob Agents Chemother 2001; 45(9): 2460–2467.

82. Moise-Broder PA, Sakoulas G, Eliopoulos GM, et al. Accessory gene regulator group II polymorphism in methicillin-resistant *Staphylococcus aureus* is predictive of failure of vancomycin therapy. Clin Infect Dis 2004; 38 (12):1700–1705.

83. Cepeda JA, Whitehouse T, Cooper B, et al. Linezolid versus teicoplanin in the treatment of Gram-positive infections in the critically ill: a randomized, double-blind, multicentre study. J Antimicrob Chemother 2004; 53(2): 345–355.

84. Sgarabotto D, Cusinato R, Narne E, et al. Synercid plus vancomycin for the treatment of severe methicillin-resistant *Staphylococcus aureus* and coagulase-negative staphylococci infections: evaluation of 5 cases. Scand J Infect Dis 2002; 34(2):122–126.

85. Anstead GM, Owens AD. Recent advances in the treatment of infections due to resistant *Staphylococcus aureus*. Curr Opin Infect Dis 2004; 17(6): 549–555.

86. Eliopoulos GM. Quinupristin-dalfopristin and linezolid: evidence and opinion. Clin Infect Dis 2003; 36(4):473–481.

87. Wunderink RG, Rello J, Cammarata SK, et al. Linezolid vs vancomycin: analysis of two double-blind studies of patients with methicillin-resistant *Staphylococcus aureus* nosocomial pneumonia. Chest 2003; 124(5): 1789–1797.

88. Kollef MH, Rello J, Cammarata SK, et al. Clinical cure and survival in Gram-positive ventilator-associated pneumonia: retrospective analysis of two double-blind studies comparing linezolid with vancomycin. Intensive Care Med 2004; 30(3):388–394.

89. Gee T, Ellis R, Marshall G, et al. Pharmacokinetics and tissue penetration of linezolid following multiple oral doses. Antimicrob Agents Chemother 2001; 45(6):1843–1846.

90. Honeybourne D, Tobin C, Jevons G, et al. Intrapulmonary penetration of linezolid. J Antimicrob Chemother 2003; 51(6):1431–1434.

91. Conte JE Jr., Golden JA, Kipps J, et al. Intrapulmonary pharmacokinetics of linezolid. Antimicrob Agents Chemother 2002; 46(5):1475–1480.

92. Boselli E, Breilh D, Rimmele T, et al. Pharmacokinetics and intrapulmonary concentrations of linezolid administered to critically ill patients with ventilator-associated pneumonia. Crit Care Med 2005; 33(7):1529–1533.

93. Bernardo K, Pakulat N, Fleer S, et al. Subinhibitory concentrations of linezolid reduce *Staphylococcus aureus* virulence factor expression. Antimicrob Agents Chemother 2004; 48(2):546–444.

94. Stevens DL, Ma Y, Salmi DB, et al. Impact of antibiotics on expression of virulence-associated exotoxin genes in methicillin-sensitive and methicillin-resistant *Staphylococcus aureus*. J Infect Dis 2007; 195(2):202–211.

95. Ohlsen K, Ziebuhr W, Koller KP, et al. Effects of subinhibitory concentrations of antibiotics on alpha-toxin (hla) gene expression of methicillin-sensitive and methicillin-resistant *Staphylococcus aureus* isolates. Antimicrob Agents Chemother 1998; 42(11):2817–2823.

96. Nasraway SA, Shorr AF, Kuter DJ, et al. Linezolid does not increase the risk of thrombocytopenia in patients with nosocomial pneumonia: comparative analysis of linezolid and vancomycin use. Clin Infect Dis 2003; 37(12): 1609–1616.

97. Shopsin B, Zhao X, Kreiswirth BN, et al. Are the new quinolones appropriate treatment for community-acquired methicillin-resistant *Staphylococcus aureus*? Int J Antimicrob Agents 2004; 24(1):32–34.

98. Hamilton-Miller JM. Reversal of activity of trimethoprim against gram-positive cocci by thymidine, thymine and "folates." J Antimicrob Chemother 1988; 22(1):35–39.

99. Pertel PE, Bernardo P, Fogarty C, et al. Effects of prior effective therapy on the efficacy of daptomycin and ceftriaxone for the treatment of community-acquired pneumonia. Clin Infect Dis 2008; 46(8):1142–1151.

100. Silverman JA, Mortin LI, Vanpraagh AD, et al. Inhibition of daptomycin by pulmonary surfactant: in vitro modeling and clinical impact. J Infect Dis 2005; 191(12):2149–2152.

101. Zhanel GG, Homenuik K, Nichol K, et al. The glycylcyclines: a comparative review with the tetracyclines. Drugs 2004; 64(1):63–88.

102. Goldstein EJ, Citron DM, Merriam CV, et al. In vitro activities of the new semisynthetic glycopeptide telavancin (TD-6424), vancomycin, daptomycin, linezolid, and four comparator agents against anaerobic gram-positive species and *Corynebacterium* spp. Antimicrob Agents Chemother 2004; 48 (6):2149–2152.

103. Reyes N, Skinner R, Kaniga K, et al. Efficacy of telavancin (TD-6424), a rapidly bactericidal lipoglycopeptide with multiple mechanisms of action, in a murine model of pneumonia induced by methicillin-resistant *Staphylococcus aureus*. Antimicrob Agents Chemother 2005; 49(10):4344–4346.

104. Fagon JY, Chastre J, Wolff M, et al. Invasive and noninvasive strategies for management of suspected ventilator-associated pneumonia. A randomized trial. Ann Intern Med 2000; 132(8):621–630.

105. Harbarth S, Dharan S, Liassine N, et al. Randomized, placebo-controlled, double-blind trial to evaluate the efficacy of mupirocin for eradicating carriage of methicillin-resistant *Staphylococcus aureus*. Antimicrob Agents Chemother 1999; 43(6):1412–1416.

106. Parras F, Guerrero MC, Bouza E, et al. Comparative study of mupirocin and oral co-trimoxazole plus topical fusidic acid in eradication of nasal carriage of methicillin-resistant *Staphylococcus aureus*. Antimicrob Agents Chemother 1995; 39(1):175–179.

107. Krueger WA, Lenhart FP, Neeser G, et al. Influence of combined intravenous and topical antibiotic prophylaxis on the incidence of infections, organ dysfunctions, and mortality in critically ill surgical patients: a prospective, stratified, randomized, double-blind, placebo-controlled clinical trial. Am J Respir Crit Care Med 2002; 166(8):1029–1037.

108. de Jonge E, Schultz MJ, Spanjaard L, et al. Effects of selective decontamination of digestive tract on mortality and acquisition of resistant bacteria in intensive care: a randomised controlled trial. Lancet 2003; 362(9389): 1011–1016.

109. Verwaest C, Verhaegen J, Ferdinande P, et al. Randomized, controlled trial of selective digestive decontamination in 600 mechanically ventilated patients in a multidisciplinary intensive care unit. Crit Care Med 1997; 25(1): 63–71.

110. Leone M, Albanese J, Antonini F, et al. Long-term (6-year) effect of selective digestive decontamination on antimicrobial resistance in intensive care, multiple-trauma patients. Crit Care Med 2003; 31(8):2090–1095.

111. Lingnau W, Berger J, Javorsky F, et al. Changing bacterial ecology during a five-year period of selective intestinal decontamination. J Hosp Infect 1998; 39(3):195–206.

112. Silvestri L, Milanese M, Oblach L, et al. Enteral vancomycin to control methicillin-resistant *Staphylococcus aureus* outbreak in mechanically ventilated patients. Am J Infect Control 2002; 30(7):391–399.

113. Bergmans DC, Bonten MJ, Gaillard CA, et al. Prevention of ventilator-associated pneumonia by oral decontamination: a prospective, randomized, double-blind, placebo-controlled study. Am J Respir Crit Care Med 2001; 164(3):382–388.

114. Pugin J, Auckenthaler R, Lew DP, et al. Oropharyngeal decontamination decreases incidence of ventilator-associated pneumonia. A randomized, placebo-controlled, double-blind clinical trial. JAMA 1991; 265(20): 2704–2710.

115. Silvestri L, van Saene HK, Milanese M, et al. Prevention of MRSA pneumonia by oral vancomycin decontamination: a randomised trial. Eur Respir J 2004; 23(6):921–926.

116. Wenisch C, Laferl H, Szell M, et al. A holistic approach to MRSA eradication in critically ill patients with MRSA pneumonia. Infection 2006; 34(3): 148–154.

Device-Related Infections and MRSA: Central Venous Catheters, Vascular Grafts, and Orthopedic Implants

Mary Beth Graham
Division of Infectious Diseases, Department of Medicine, Medical College of Wisconsin, Milwaukee, Wisconsin, U.S.A.

INTRODUCTION

A variety of implantable medical devices have been developed to improve the health and well-being of patients and can be used on either a short-term [e.g., urinary catheter, central venous catheter (CVC)] or permanent (e.g., orthopedic implant, vascular graft prosthesis) basis. These medical devices are made from biomaterials, which are inert, nonviable materials intended to interact with biologic systems to perform, augment, or replace a natural function (1). Despite the improved quality of life that these biomaterials can offer, it has been reported that approximately half of the two million cases of nosocomial infections that occur each year in the United States are associated with indwelling devices (2).

The incidence of prosthetic device infections varies with the type of implant. The highest rates of infection occur with left ventricular assist devices with rates of 50% or greater. Orthopedic implants are reported to have among the lowest rates, with infection occurring in <1% of initial total hip arthroplastic procedures and <2% of initial total knee arthroplasties (3). Rates of infection tend to be greater after revision than after primary device implantation. This greater rate of infection has been attributed to a number of factors, including impaired circulation as a result of scarring from the previous procedure and longer operating times involved in revision surgeries (4).

Staphylococci, particularly coagulase-negative staphylococci, are ubiquitous inhabitants of the skin and mucous membranes, and the predominant organisms implicated in most device-related infections (4,5). Colonization with coagulase-positive staphylococci, either MSSA or MRSA, has also been implicated as a potential risk factor for subsequent infection with these organisms (6,7). Staphylococcal organisms on the skin, incisional margins, hair follicles, sweat glands, and lymphatic structures are all potential sources for device contamination either at the time of surgery by direct contamination or afterward when organisms can reach the device either through lymphatics or hematogenously. In addition to host colonization, the type of material used and the construction of the device may contribute to the overall risk of infection (8). *Staphylococcus aureus* is a major pathogen associated with metallic implants, whereas *S. epidermidis* and *Pseudomonas* are isolated more frequently from polymeric implants. For all organisms associated with implant infections, the course of infection involves three major steps: (*i*) microbial adhesion to the implant, (*ii*) microbial proliferation, and (*iii*) formation of a bacterial biofilm. Staphylococcal biolfilms and their potential role in maintaining colonization and avoiding action of host immune factors and antibiotics were first reported in 1972 (9), and research in this area remains active to this day.

This chapter will concentrate on the three areas: (*i*) the pathogenesis of prosthetic device infections focusing on biofilm formation and function; (*ii*) the incidence and risk factors for three types of implantable devices in which infection with staphylococcal organisms, including MRSA, play a significant role in the morbidity and mortality; and (*iii*) the prevention and treatment options for device-related infections.

THE IMPORTANCE OF BIOFILMS

A biofilm is a complex structured community of microorganisms encapsulated within a self-developed polymeric matrix and adherent to a living or inert surface. After insertion of a prosthetic device, a layer of plasma proteins, such as fibronectin, fibrinogen, and collagen, form a surface on the device to which free-floating, or planktonic, bacteria can adhere (10). This host-derived layer is especially important, as some organisms, such as *S. aureus* and several species of *Streptococcus*, have fibronectin receptors that increase their ability to adhere to both native tissues and foreign bodies and augment the formation of biofilms (11). Once bacteria have adhered to the surface of the device, they multiply and produce extracellular glycoproteins that form a glycocalyx in which the bacteria become attached to one another and promote spread over the surface of the device. As this bacterial layer develops, the bacteria slow their rate of growth and become resistant to innate host defenses, such as antibodies and phagocytic cells. Biofilm bacteria also become more resistant to antimicrobial agents. It is estimated that bacteria in biofilms are 10 to 1000 times more resistant to antibiotics than their planktonic counterparts (12). A specific behavior change that has been reported for *S. aureus* is the formation small-colony variants (SCVs), which have reduced growth rates and increased resistance to aminoglycosides and cell wall–active antibiotics (13). Their slow growth rate raises a challenge for the microbiology laboratory, as these variants may not be recovered with standard culture techniques. *S. aureus* SCVs and planktonic bacteria have the same appearance on Gram staining, but SCVs grow 2^9 times more slowly than do their planktonic counterparts and often have decreased coagulase activity, which may lead to misidentification. As seen with other biofilm-associated bacteria, the MICs of antibiotics for SCVs are often beyond clinically achievable levels. These organisms have been referred to as "Trojan horses," as SCVs are able to persist and hide within host phagocytic cells, such as fibroblasts and endothelial cells, where they are protected from host defenses and exposure to antibiotics. However, after discontinuation of antibiotic therapy, they can revert to their planktonic, more virulent forms with resultant signs and symptoms of recurrent infection for the patient.

The mechanism that mediates the change in behavior from free-living planktonic forms to biofilm-associated bacteria is regulated by quorum sensing via the accessory gene regulator (*agr*) system (11,14,15). The *agr* system influences cell-to-cell communication and regulation of growth and virulence factors and is thought to play a significant role in the chronic nature of *S. aureus* and *S. epidermidis* biofilm-associated infections. The staphylococcal *agr* quorum-sensing system decreases the expression of several cell surface proteins and increases expression of many secreted virulence factors. The quorum response in staphylococci during an infection occurs within a complex regulatory network of other gene products that continually modifies either *agr* activity itself or its downstream effects (14). Dysfunction in *agr* is associated with persistent bacteremia with MRSA and appears more commonly in disease-causing staphylococcal organisms, as opposed to colonizing isolates, raising the possibility that such strains may be selected nosocomially (16,17). Loss of function of *agr* is also associated with the emergence of glyco-peptide intermediate *S. aureus*, which leads to treatment failures with vancomycin (18).

BIOFILMS AND ANTIBIOTICS

Antibiotic therapy often alleviates the signs and symptoms of infection associated with implanted devices by killing the planktonic bacteria that are released from the biofilm in a natural pattern of programmed detachment. However, this same antibiotic therapy alone often fails to kill the sessile organisms in the biofilm or fully eradicate the source of infection (10,19). The mechanisms by which biofilms confer resistance to antimicrobial agents are multifactorial and include delayed penetration of antimicrobial agents through the biofilm matrix, altered growth of biofilm bacteria, and inability of host defense mechanisms to destroy biofilm microorganisms. One of the most active antibiotics against biofilm-associated staphylococcal organisms is rifampin (20,21). Rifampin is able to penetrate through the biofilm matrix and is bactericidal against slow-growing and adherent staphylococcal organisms; however, resistance develops quickly if this agent is used alone. On the basis of these findings, current medical therapy for MRSA device-related infections typically includes rifampin combined with an agent active against MRSA. Vancomycin or teicoplanin in combination with rifampin have been studied most extensively for the treatment of MRSA prosthetic infections and are still considered the treatments of choice, although treatment failures occur. On the basis of a recent study, it might be prudent to use an MRSA active agent other than vancomycin if the MRSA isolate has an elevated vancomycin MIC (22). Patients with MRSA bacteremia with a vancomycin MIC $\geq$ 1.5 responded poorly to vancomycin treatment, regardless of the trough level achieved (22). These results apply to MRSA infection and should not be generalized to other staphylococcal organisms. Numerous reports document favorable outcomes when combining rifampin with daptomycin, linezolid, fluoroquinolones, quinupristin-dalfopristin, trimethoprim-sulfamethoxazole, clindamycin, or tetracycline/glycylcycline antibiotics (13,19,21,23–25). However, no single combination has been proven consistently superior to other combinations for the treatment of MRSA device-related infections.

CENTRAL VENOUS CATHETER INFECTIONS

Intravascular access catheters are essential medical devices that are routinely used in health care settings. In the United States, health care institutions purchase millions of intravascular catheters and estimated use in intensive care units (ICUs) is approximately 15 million catheter days annually (26). Intravascular devices are the single most important cause of health care–associated blood stream infections, with an estimated 250,000 to 500,000 infections occurring annually in the United States (27). Coagulase-negative staphylococci followed by *S. aureus* and

Enterococcus are the most frequently reported causes of catheter-related blood stream infections (CR-BSIs), accounting for 37%, 13%, and 13% of CR-BSI's, respectively (26). It is estimated that up to 50% of *S. aureus* CR-BSI's are caused by MRSA, and may be even higher in certain patient populations, specifically those on hemodialysis (28).

Pooled mean rates for all CR-BSI in U.S. hospitals ranged from 0.5 to 5.6 infections per 1000 catheter days (29). For MRSA, the pooled mean number of CR-BSI per 1000 device days ranged from 0.18 to the highest rate of 0.93 in burn ICUs (30). Overall, a CR-BSI can increase health care costs significantly, ranging from $4000 to $56,000 per episode (27). MRSA CR-BSIs significantly increased the cost of hospitalization compared to MSSA CR-BSIs with median hospital charges of $26,424 versus $19,212 (31). These costs become increasingly significant because the Centers for Medicare and Medicaid Services (CMS) will no longer reimburse a hospital at a higher rate for vascular catheter–associated infections acquired while in the hospital (32).

The majority of CR-BSIs are associated with the use of surgically implanted cuffed and tunneled all-purpose CVCs (27). A CR-BSI is defined as bacteremia/fungemia in a patient with an intravascular catheter with at least one positive blood culture obtained from a peripheral vein, clinical manifestations of infection (i.e., fever, chills, and/or hypotension), and no apparent source of the BSI except the catheter.

One of the following should also be present:

1. An yield of >15 CFU from a catheter by semiquantitative means or an yield of $>10^2$ CFU from a catheter by quantitative means with the same organism (species and antibiogram) isolated from the catheter segment and peripheral blood
2. Simultaneous quantitative blood cultures with a >5:1 ratio CVC versus peripheral
3. Differential period of CVC culture versus peripheral blood culture positivity of less than two hours (26)

An MRSA CR-BSI is suspected in any patient with risk factors for MRSA and central venous access. Reported risk factors for MRSA CR-BSIs include recent exposure to a health care setting (especially hospitalization period in an ICU), residence in a long-term care facility, presence of an open wound, exposure to antibiotics, and nasal carriage of MRSA (6,33,34). A positive blood culture for MRSA, clinical signs and symptoms, and a CVC increases the suspicion for an MRSA CR-BSI. The absence of any other identifiable source for infection confirms the diagnosis. The mortality rate attributed to catheter-related *S. aureus* bacteremia (8.2%) significantly exceeds the mortality rate for coagulase-negative staphylococcal CR-BSI (0.7%) (35).

Management of an MRSA CR-BSI varies according to the type of catheter involved. A nontunneled catheter should be removed and the tip cultured. Often it is not feasible to remove these lines initially, especially if the patient has limited venous access options and/or the line is being used for hemodialysis or chemotherapy. The decision-making process about whether to remove the line should include an assessment of the severity of the patient's illness and presence of complications, such as endocarditis, septic thrombosis, tunnel infection, or metastatic seeding (35). If not contraindicated, it is recommended that a transesophageal echocardiogram (TEE) be done to rule out vegetations in patients with *S. aureus* CR-BSI, as endocarditis is documented in up to 23% of patients with apparently uncomplicated *S. aureus* CR-BSI (36).

The most recent guidelines for the prevention of CR-BSI were published in 2009, which recommend that the preferred treatment for MRSA CR-BSI is vancomycin (37). If the MIC of the isolate is >1.5 μg/mL, daptomycin at a dose of 6 mg/kg/day should be considered (22). Linezolid, trimethoprim-sulfamethoxazole, or vancomycin plus rifampin or gentamicin are listed as alternative therapies for proven cases of MRSA CR-BSI. Duration of therapy for *S. aureus* CR-BSI depends on whether the infection is considered uncomplicated or complicated and whether the line is removed or left in place. For nontunneled catheters and tunneled catheters that can be removed, patients are started on appropriate antibiotics and the line removed. After removal, repeat peripheral blood cultures are drawn. If those cultures are negative and the patient responds rapidly to therapy, the patient can be treated with antibiotics for two weeks. If blood cultures remain positive after removal of the line, a TEE should be performed. If the TEE is positive, the patient remains on therapy for four to six weeks and has blood cultures drawn on a daily basis until negative. If the TEE is negative, a search for an alternate source of the bacteremia is undertaken.

For tunneled catheters that must be retained, a TEE is ordered to assess for endocarditis. If positive, the line is removed and the patient treated for four to six weeks with appropriate antibiotics. If the TEE is negative and there is no evidence of complications or tunnel infection, the patient is treated with four weeks of systemic antibiotics plus antibiotic lock therapy. This recommendation is specifically for *S. aureus* CR-BSI, noting that antibiotic lock is not routinely recommended for MRSA CR-BSI unless there is no alternative catheter insertion site available. If lock therapy is used, dwell times for the antibiotic solution should not exceed 48 hours before reinstallation. For vancomycin, the concentration used in the lock solution should be at least 1000 times higher than the MIC (e.g., 5 mg/mL). If there is relapsing or persistent bacteremia, or if the patient deteriorates, the catheter should be removed. In addition, patients with evidence of metastatic disease, such as osteomyelitis or abscesses, should have the line removed and be treated with systemic antibiotics for six to eight weeks (35).

In 2002, CDC published evidence-based guidelines for the prevention of intravascular catheter-related infections (38). Strategies proposed include quality assurance and continuing education, selection of site of catheter insertion (e.g., choosing sites with lower densities of skin flora), hand hygiene and aseptic technique, use of antimicrobial/antiseptic impregnated catheters and cuffs, use of antibiotic/antiseptic ointments at the insertion site, antibiotic lock prophylaxis, and scheduled replacement of nontunneled IV catheters and IV administration sets. Antimicrobial-impregnated catheter is a strategy that has variable efficacy. An excellent review evaluating the efficacy of chlorhexidine-silver sulfadiazine- or minocycline-rifampin-impregnated CVCs was published by Crnich and Maki in 2004 (39). They did not recommend the routine use of anti-microbial impregnated CVCs because of their substantial cost. They did recommend the use of these catheters where rates of CR-BSI remain high ($\geq$3.3 BSIs per 1000 catheter days) despite consistent and appropriate use of infection control practices.

Other authors have suggested additional interventions to prevent the development of CR-BSIs. Nasal carriage of *S. aureus* is thought to be a risk factor of development of bacteremia, and the highest prevalence of carriage appears to occur among dialysis patients with rates as high as 60% (7,28,35). One intriguing study showed that use of nasal mupirocin led to eradication of nasal *S. aureus* carriage in 96.3% of surveillance cultures and a fourfold reduction in the incidence of *S. aureus* bacteremia per patient-year in hemodialysis patients (40). However, emergence of resistance to mupirocin in MRSA isolates often develops after use, thus limiting the broad applicability of this practice (41).

VASCULAR GRAFT INFECTIONS

Prosthetic vascular grafts are classified as either biologic or synthetic. Biologic grafts can either be autografts or allografts and are typically used in peripheral vascular surgical procedures and in coronary artery bypass procedures. Synthetic grafts are commonly made from dacron or poly-tetrafluoroethylene and are used for hemodialysis access and aortic or aortoiliac surgeries. Infection rates of vascular grafts vary with the type of graft. Hemodialysis arteriovenous grafts have an infection rate of >5%. Femoropopliteal grafts have an infection rate of approximately 4%. The lowest rate of infection occurs with aortic grafts (2%), but these infections have the highest rates of morbidity and mortality (2,42). The major risk factors for developing a vascular surgical site infection and possibly a graft infection are nasal carriage of MSSA or MRSA, recent hospitalization, failed arterial reconstruction, and presence of a groin incision (43).

Grafts become infected secondary to contamination at the time of insertion, migration of organisms from the overlying skin, or via lymphangitic or hematogenous spread. *S. aureus*, *S. epidermidis*, and *Escherichia coli* currently account for up to 75% of graft infections (44). The incidence of MRSA infections in vascular surgery patients has risen steadily over the past 10 years in the United States and in Europe, and in some institutions accounts for over 50% of the vascular graft infections seen (43). MRSA vascular graft infections are associated with increased risk of amputation, increased risk of death (odds ratio 3.4 compared to MSSA), and prolonged hospitalizations.

The diagnostic criteria for a vascular graft infection include signs/symptoms of infection at the graft site including pain, tenderness, erythema, and swelling. The presence of perigraft fluid or perigraft soft-tissue swelling beyond three months or perigraft air beyond four to seven weeks is considered abnormal and suspicious for infection. CT scanning is the preferred diagnostic imaging modality and it is used to guide aspiration of any fluid collections found (44). Purulent drainage and organisms isolated from aseptically obtained cultures of fluid or tissue secures the diagnosis of a vascular graft infection.

Treatment of a vascular graft infection is surgical with intravenous antibiotics chosen on the basis of culture results. The surgical procedure chosen depends on the type of graft and the condition of the patient. Graft salvage is considered for some vascular graft infections, but should not be considered when the infecting organism is MRSA (45). Regardless of procedure, culture-specific intravenous antibiotics are used perioperatively and postoperatively for up to six weeks especially if the infection is associated with bacteremia or an abscess. Biofilms form in vascular grafts and add to the pathogenesis of the infection. A combination of rifampin with vancomycin, teichoplanin, daptomycin, or linezolid should be used to cover gram-positive organisms including MRSA. For initial empiric therapy, these medications should be combined with a β-lactam antibiotic, or aztreonam if the patient is allergic to penicillin or cephalosporin, to cover potential gram-negative organisms.

Strategies to prevent vascular graft infections are similar to those employed to prevent CR-BSIs. They include patient screening for nasal carriage of *Staphylococcus* (both MRSA and MSSA) and decolonization with nasal mupirocin if positive, as well as fastidious attention to hand hygiene and barrier precautions. Removal of operative site hair at the time of operation using clippers rather than a razor and skin preparation with 10% providone-iodine or chlorhexidine gluconate will help prevent carriage of skin flora in the wound (44). Strategies employed by some surgeons have also included soaking gelatin-coated polyester or polytetrafluoroethylene vascular prostheses in rifampin (30–60 mg/mL) solution prior to implantation and using silver-impregnated wound dressings for postoperative femoral/groin incision care. In addition to standard perioperative prophylactic antibiotic treatment with cefazolin or cefuroxime, intravenous vancomycin or daptomycin is added for patients considered at high risk for an MRSA postoperative infection for a total of 24 hours (43).

ORTHOPEDIC IMPLANT INFECTIONS

The number of knee and hip replacement surgeries has increased steadily worldwide, and it is estimated that the demand for primary total knee and hip arthroplasties will grow by 673% and 174%, respectively, by the year 2030 (46). The infection rates after primary knee and hip replacement are low, estimated at <2% internationally and <1 % in the United States (47,48). Infection rates after revision surgery are considerably higher, with estimates at 40% (49). Orthopedic device-related infections (ODRIs) are typically classified as early (<3 months postsurgery), late chronic (3–24 months postsurgery), or hematogenous. Coagulase-positive staphylococci are primary pathogens in all three categories, especially within the first three months postoperatively (47,49). The formation of a biofilm on the surface of the orthopedic prosthesis is an essential factor in the development and persistence of infection.

Diagnosis of an ODRI includes evaluation of the clinical presentation and review of laboratory, histopathology, microbiology, and radiographic studies. Typically, patients will present with pain at the site of the device and variably with erythema, warmth, and swelling over the joint in question. Blood leukocyte count and differential may or may not be elevated. ESR and CRP are elevated in a majority of patients with ODRIs (50). Analysis of synovial fluid leukocyte count and differential is a simple way to differentiate prosthetic joint-associated infection from aseptic failure. A synovial fluid leukocyte count of $>1.7 \times 10^9$/L and a differential of $>65\%$ neutrophils has a sensitivity of 94% to 97% and a specificity of 88% to 98% for infection. *S. aureus* is often associated with leukocyte counts $>100 \times 10^3$/mL (51). Acute inflammation in the periprosthetic tissue is useful in establishing the diagnosis of an ODRI (49). Preoperative aspiration of the joint and at least three intraoperative tissue cultures should be obtained when considering the diagnosis of an ODRI. If possible, the patient should be off all antibiotics at least two weeks prior to tissue sampling and some authors recommend preoperative antibiotics not be started until after tissue specimens are collected (47,49). Periprosthetic lucencies with evidence of bone resorption on radiograph or loosening of the prosthesis raise the suspicion for the presence of infection (52).

Surgical intervention and prolonged antimicrobial therapy are necessary to treat an ODRI. A two-stage procedure involving removal of the infected prosthesis and associated foreign material, placement of an antibiotic-loaded acrylic cement spacer, and treatment with approximately six weeks of intravenous antibiotics followed by reimplantation is a common strategy with success rates of $\geq 90\%$ (53,54). This approach is primarily used for late chronic infections. Early postoperative infections and acute hematogenous infections are treated by debriding infected tissue, retaining the prosthesis and prolonged intravenous antibiotic therapy with success rates up to 80%. Failure rates increase when there is a sinus tract, symptoms prior to debridement ≥8 days, underlying comorbidities such as rheumatoid arthritis and diabetes mellitus, and *S. aureus* as the etiologic agent (55). Since failure is increased with *S. aureus*, many orthopedic surgeons favor the two-stage revision for MRSA ODRIs (47).

The current recommended treatment for MRSA ODRIs is vancomcyin plus rifampin for four to eight weeks post removal of the prosthesis and placement of an antibiotic-impregnated spacer. Gentamicin and tobramycin are the most common antimicrobials impregnated into polymethylmethacrylate used in spacers for two-stage revisions. However, MSSA is often resistant to gentamicin (29%) and tobramycin (46%), and up to 100% MRSA isolates are resistant to tobramycin (56). The patient is then monitored off antibiotic therapy for one to two months prior to reimplantation of the joint prosthesis.

Debridement and retention of an MRSA-infected prosthesis, followed by prolonged suppressive antibiotic therapy, are associated with variable success (55,57). If this surgical option is chosen, the initial treatment should include intravenous vancomycin plus rifampin for six to eight weeks, followed by oral therapy. Alternate initial agents include daptomycin and linezolid, both of which eradicate adherence of staphylococcal organisms in vitro from prosthetic devices (19). Oral agents used for prolonged suppressive therapy include ciprofloxacin, trimethoprim-sulfamethoxazole, minocycline, or doxycycline combined with rifampin (47,49,57).

Preventative measures for MRSA ODRIs have focused on decreasing MRSA colonization on the skin by using topical chlorhexidine and intranasal mupirocin. Despite conflicting results regarding the efficacy of intranasal mupirocin in reducing the risk of postoperative infections, many orthopedic programs, including ours, have instituted programs of preoperative screening for nasal carriage of MRSA. If positive, intranasal mupirocin is prescribed and vancomcyin is used for perioperative prophylaxis instead of a cephalosporin (58–61). Additional studies are needed to assess whether alternative agents, such as linezolid or daptomycin, should be used routinely for perioperative prophylaxis in patients at risk for postoperative infection with MRSA.

SUMMARY

MRSA is an important pathogen in device-related infections, in part because of its ability to form a biofilm on the surface of the implanted foreign body. It is associated with increased morbidity and mortality as well as hospital costs. Strategies to reduce the number of MRSA device-related infections include fastidious adherence to infection control guidelines and interventions to decrease skin and nasal colonization. When infections occur, removal of the infected material combined with antibiotic therapy is the most definitive approach to treatment. However, salvage of the infected prosthesis can potentially be achieved through surgical debridement and appropriate antibiotic therapy.

REFERENCES

1. William DF. Review: Tissue-biomaterial interactions. J Mat Sci 1987; 22:3421–3445.
2. Darouiche RO. Treatment of infections associated with surgical implants. N Engl J Med 2004; 350:1422–1429.
3. Zimmerli W, Trampuz A, Ochsner PE. Prosthetic joint infections. N Engl J Med 2004; 351:1645–1654.
4. Sampedro MF, Patel R. Infections associated with long-term prosthetic devices. Infect Dis Clin N Am 2007; 21:785–819.
5. Edmiston CE. Infections of prosthetic devices in surgery. In: Nylus LM, ed. Problems in General Surgery: Surgical Sepsis 1993 and Beyond. Vol. 10, Issue 3. Philadelphia: JB Lippincott Company, 1993:444–468.
6. Coello R, Glynn JR, Gaspar C, et al. Risk Factors for developing clinical infections with methicillin-resistant *Staphylococcus aureus* (MRSA) amongst

hospital patients initially colonized with MRSA. J Hosp Infect 1997; 37(1): 39–46.

7. Huang SS, Platt R. Risk of methicillin-resistant *Staphylococcus aureus* infection after previous infection or colonization. Clin Infect Dis 2003; 36:281–285.

8. Maathuis PGM, Bulstra SK, van der Mei HC, et al. Biomaterial-associated surgery and infection: a review of literature. In: Rakhorst G, Ploeg R, eds. Biomaterials in Modern Medicine: The Groningen Perspective. Vol. 7. Singapore: World Scientific, 2008:119–138.

9. Bayston R, Penny SR. Excessive production of mucoid substance in staphylococcus SIIA: a possible factor in colonization of holter shunts. Dev Med Child Neurol 1972; 14S:25–28.

10. Costerton JS, Stewart PS, Greenberg EP. Bacterial biofilms: a common cause of persistent infections. Science 1999; 284:1318–1322.

11. Donlan, RM, Costerton, JW. Biofilms: survival mechanisms of clinically relevant microorganisms. Clin Microbiol Rev 2002; 15:167–193.

12. Widmer AF, Frei R, Rajacic Z, et al. Correlation between in vivo and in vitro efficacy of antimicrobial agents against foreign body infections. J Infect Dis 1990; 162:96–102.

13. Proctor RA, Peters G. Small colony variants in staphylococcal infections: diagnostic and therapeutic implications. Clin Infect Dis 1998; 2:419–423.

14. Yarwood JM, Schlievert PM. Quorum sensing in *Staphylococcus* infections. J Clin Invest 2003; 112(11):1620–1625.

15. Novick RP, Geisinger E. Quorum sensing in staphylococci. Annu Rev Genet 2008; 42:541–564.

16. Fowler VG Jr., Sakoulas G, McIntyre LM, et al. Persistent bacteremia due to methicillin-resistant *Staphylococcus aureus* infection is associated with *agr* dysfunction and low-level in vitro resistance to thrombin-induced platelet microbicidal protein. J Infect Dis 2004; 190:1140–1149.

17. Shopsin B, Drlica-Wagner A, Mathema B, et al. Prevalence of *agr* dysfunction among colonizing *Staphylococcus aureus* strains. J Infect Dis 2008; 198:1171–1174.

18. Salkoulas G, Eliopoulos GM, Fowler VG Jr., et al. Reduced susceptibility of *Staphylococcus aureus* to vancomycin and platelet microbicidal protein correlates with defective autolysis and loss of accessory gene regulator (*agr*) function. Antimicrob Agents Chemother 2005; 49(7):2687–2692.

19. Edmiston CE, Goheen MP, Seabrook GR, et al. Impact of selective antimicrobial agents on staphylococcal adherence to biomedical devices. Am J Surg 2006; 192:344–354.

20. Monzon M, Oteiza C, Leiva J, et al. Synergy of different antibiotic combinations in biofilms of *Staphylococcus epidermidis*. J Antimicrob Chemother 2001; 48:793–801.

21. Saginur R, St. Denis M, Ferris W, et al. Multiple combination bactericidal testing of staphylococcal biofilms from implant-associated infections. Antimicrob Agents Chemother 2006; 50(1):55–61.

22. Lodise TP, Graves J, Evans A, et al. Relationship between vancomycin MIC and failure among patients with MRSA bacteremia treated with vancomycin. Antimicrob Agents Chemother 2008; 52(9):3315–3320.

23. Lentino JR, Narita M, Yu VL. New antimicrobial agents as therapy for resistant gram-positive Cocci. Eur J Clin Microbiol Infect Dis 2008; 27: 3–15.

24. Rose WE, Poppens PT. Impact of biofilms on the in vitro activity of vancomycin alone and in combination with tigecycline and rifampicin against *Staphylococcus aureus*. J Antimicrob Chemother 2009; 63(3):485–488.

25. Smith K, Perez A, Ramage G, et al. Comparison of biofilm-associated cell survival following in vitro exposure of methicillin-resistant *Staphylococcus aureus* biofilms to the antibiotics clindamycin, daptomycin, linezolid, tigecycline, and vancomycin. Int J Antimicrob Agents 2009; 33(4):374–378.

26. O'Grady NP, Alexander M, Dellinger EP, et al. Guidelines for the prevention of intravascular catheter-related infections. Pediatrics 2002; 110(5):e51. Available at: http://www.pediatrics.org/cgi/content/full/110/5/e51.

27. Maki DF, Kluger DM, Crnich CJ. The risk of bloodstream infection in adults with different intravascular devices: a systematic review of 200 published prospective studies. Mayo Clin Proc 2006; 81(9):1159–1171.

28. Reed SD, Friedman JY, Engemann JJ, et al. Costs and outcomes among hemodialysis-dependent patients with methicillin-resistant or methicillin-susceptible *Staphylococcus aureus* bacteremia. Infect Control Hosp Epidemiol 2005; 26:175–183.

29. Edwards JR, Peterson KD, Andrus ML, et al. National Healthcare Safety Network (NHSN) Report, data summary for 2006 through 2007, issued November 2008. Am J Infect Control 2008; 36:609–626.

30. Hidron AI, Edwards JR, Patel J, et al. Antimicrobial-resistant pathogens associated with healthcare-associated infections: annual summary of data reported to the national healthcare safety network at the centers for disease control and prevention, 2006–2007. Infect Control Hosp Epidemiol 2008; 29(11):996–1011.

31. Cosgrove SE, Qi Y, Kaye KS, et al. The Impact of methicillin resistance in *Staphylococcus aureus* bacteremia on patient outcomes: mortality, length of stay, and hospital charges. Infect Control Hosp Epidemiol 2005; 26:166–174.

32. CMS Press Release April 14, 2008. Available at: http://www.cms.hhs.gov.

33. Von Eiff C, Becker K, Machka K, et al. Nasal carriage as a source of *Staphylococcus aureus* bacteremia. N Engl J Med 2001; 344(1):11–16.

34. Oztoprak N, Cevik MA, Akinci E, et al. Risk factors for ICU-acquired methicillin-resistant *Staphylococcus aureus* infection. Am J Infect Control 2006; 34(1):1–5.

35. Mermel LA, Farr BM, Sherertz RJ, et al. Guidelines for the management of intravascular catheter-related infections. Clin Infect Dis 2001; 32:1249–1272.

36. Rosen AB, Fowler VG, Corey GR, et al. Cost-effectiveness of trans-esophageal echocardiography to determine the duration of therapy for intravascular catheter–associated *Staphylococcus aureus* bacteremia. Ann Intern Med 1999; 130(10):810–820.

37. Mermel LA, Allon M, Bouza E, et al. Clinical practice guidelines for the diagnosis and management of intravascular catheter-related infection: 2009 update by the infectious diseases society of America. Clin Infect Dis 2009; 49:1–45.

38. Guidelines for the prevention of intravascular catheter-related infections. MMWR 2002; 51: No.RR-10. Available at: http://www.cdc.gov/mmwr/PDF/rr/rr5110.pdf.

39. Crnich CJ, Maki DG. Are antimicrobial-impregnated catheters effective? Don't throw out the baby with the bathwater. Clin Infect Dis 2004; 38: 1287–1292.

40. Boelaert JR, Van Landuyt HW, Godard CA, et al. Nasal mupirocin ointment decreases the incidence of *Staphylococcus aureus* bacteremias in haemo-dialysis patients. Nephrol Dial Transplant 1993; 8:235–239.

41. Miller MA, Dascal A, Portnoy J, et al. Development of mupirocin resistance among methicillin-resistant *Staphylococcus aureus* after widespread use of nasal mupirocin ointment. Infect Control Hosp Epidemiol 1996; 17:811–813.

42. Perea GB, Fujitani RM, Kubaska SM. Aortic graft infection: update on management and treatment options. Vasc Endovascular Surg 2006; 40:1–10.

43. Bandyk DF. Vascular surgical site infection: risk factors and preventive measures. Semin Vasc Surg 2008; 21:119–123.

44. Herscu G, Wilson SE. Prosthetic infection: lessons from treatment of the infected vascular graft. Surg Clin N Am 2009; 89:391–401.

45. Zetrenne E, McIntosh BC, McRae MH, et al. Prosthetic vascular graft infection: a multi-center review of surgical management. Yale J Biol Med 2007; 20:113–121.
46. Kurtz S, Ong K, Lau E, et al. Projections of primary and revision hip and knee arthroplasty in the united states from 2005 to 2030. J Bone Joint Surg Am 2007; 89(4):780–785.
47. Widmer, AF. New developments in diagnosis and treatment of infection in orthopedic implants. Clin Infect Dis 2001; 33(suppl 2):S94–S106.
48. Kurtz SM, Lau E, Schmler J, et al. Infection burden for hip and knee arthroplasty in the United States. J Arthroplasty 2008; 23(7):984–991.
49. Trampuz A, Widmer AF. Infections associated with orthopedic implants. Curr Opin Infect Dis 2006; 19:349–356.
50. Austin MS, Ghanem E, Joshi A, et al. A simple, cost-effective screening protocol to rule out periprosthetic infection. J Arthroplasty 2008; 23(1):65–68.
51. Trampuz a, Hanssen AD, Osmon DR, et al. Synovial fluid leukocyte count and differential for the diagnosis of prosthetic knee infection. Am J Med 2004; 117:556–562.
52. Levine SE, Esterhai JL Jr., Heppenstall RB, et al. Diagnoses and staging. Osteomyelitis and prosthetic joint infections. Clin Orthop Relat Res 1993; 295:77–86.
53. Haddad FS, Masri BA, Campbell D, et al. The PROSTALAC functional spacer in two-stage revision for infected knee replacements. J Bone Joint Surg Br 2000; 82(6):807–812.
54. Cui Q, Mihalko WM, Shields JS, et al. Antibiotic-impregnated cement spacers for the treatment of infection associated with total hip or knee arthoplasty. J Bone Joint Surg Am 2007; 89:871–82.
55. Marculescu CE, Berbari EF, Hanssen AD, et al. Outcome of prosthetic joint infections treated with debridement and retention of components. Clin Infect Dis 2006; 42:471–478.
56. Anguita-Alonso P, Hanssen AD, Osmon DR, et al. High rate of amino-glycoside resistance among staphylococci causing prosthetic joint infection. Clin Orthop Relat Res 2005; 439:43–47.
57. Segreti J, Nelson JA, Tenholme GM. Prolonged suppressive antibiotic therapy for infected orthopedic prostheses. Clin Infect Dis 1998; 27:711–713.
58. Kalmeijer MD, Coertjens H, van Nieuwland-Bollen M, et al. Surgical site infections in orthopedic surgery: the effect of mupirocin nasal ointment in a double-blind, randomized, placebo controlled study. Clin Infect Dis 2002; 35:353–358.

59. Wilcox MH, Hall J, Pike H, et al. Use of perioperative mupirocin to prevent methicillin-resistant *Staphylococcus aureus* (MRSA) orthopaedic surgical site infections. J Hosp Infect 2003; 54:196–201.
60. de Lucas-Villarrubia JC, Lopez-Franco M, Granizo JJ, et al. Strategy to control methicillin-resistant *Staphylococcus aureus* post-operative infection in orthopaedic surgery. Int Orthop 2004; 28:16–20.
61. Sanderson PJ. The role of methicillin-resistant *Staphylococcus aureus* in orthopaedic implant surgery. J Chemother 2001; 13:89–95.

MRSA Bacteremia

Melissa Brunsvold and Lena M. Napolitano
Department of Surgery, University of Michigan Health System, Ann Arbor,
Michigan, U.S.A.

NOSOCOMIAL BACTEREMIA AND MRSA

Bacteremia is the third most common nosocomial infection, with urinary tract infection most common, and pneumonia ranking second (1,2). The most common causative pathogens for bacteremia are gram-positive pathogens, accounting for 65% of cases, including coagulase-negative staphylococci and *Staphylococcus aureus* (Table 1). The SCOPE project examined 24,179 cases of nosocomial bacteremia in 49 U.S. hospitals between 1995 and 2002, and documented a 10% increase in bacteremia due to gram-positive cocci, with a concomitant 10% decrease in the percentage of bacteremia due to gram-negative bacilli (from 33.2% in 1986 to 23.8% in 2003) (4). *S. aureus* was the second most common bacteremia isolate after coagulase-negative staphylococci, accounting for 20% of cases. Most important, the proportion of methicillin-resistant *S. aureus* (MRSA) bacteremia isolates increased from 22% in 1995 to 57% in 2001 (3). In intensive care unit (ICU) patients, 59.5% of all *S. aureus* isolates associated with nosocomial infections are now methicillin resistant (5). In a U.S. study by the Surveillance Network, annual rates of MRSA were shown to have increased steadily during 1998–2005, with rates of up to 59.2% among *S. aureus* isolates in clinical specimens from non-ICU patients. In the same study, MRSA constituted 49.1% of bloodstream *S. aureus* isolates from inpatients and 41.4% of such isolates from outpatients (6). Overall rates of *S. aureus* bacteremia are on the rise; this is due to a significant increase in the rates of MRSA bacteremia.

TABLE 1 Most Common Nosocomial Bacteremia Pathogens in the United States

Rank	Pathogen	Percent of all bacteremia isolates	Mortality (%)
1	Coagulase-negative staphylococci	31.3	20.7
2	*Staphylococcus aureus*	20.2	25.4
3	*Enterococcus* spp.	9.4	33.9
4	*Candida* spp.	9.0	39.2
5	*Escherichia coli*	5.6	22.4
6	*Klebsiella* spp.	4.8	27.6
7	*Pseudomonas aeruginosa*	4.3	38.7
8	*Enterobacter* spp.	3.9	26.7
9	*Serratia* spp.	1.7	27.4
10	*Acinetobacter baumannii*	1.3	34.0

Source: From Ref. 3.

Initial MRSA clinical isolates were reported in the United States as early as the 1960s, shortly after the introduction of methicillin in 1959 (7). Resistance to methicillin is defined as an oxacillin minimum inhibitory concentration (MIC) of 4 mg/mL. Isolates that are methicillin resistant are resistant to all β-lactams. Antibiotic resistance is mediated by the *mec* gene on a sequence called the staphylococcal chromosomal cassette (SCC*mec*). There have been five types of SCC*mec* identified. Types I to III are associated with hospital-acquired MRSA and are multidrug resistant. Type IV is associated with community-associated MRSA (CA-MRSA) and has a more favorable antibiotic susceptibility pattern.

MRSA VS. MSSA BACTEREMIA AND OUTCOMES

Mortality is high in hospitalized patients who develop MRSA bacteremia with reported short-term mortality rates of 12% to 35%. There is general consensus in the published literature that MRSA bacteremia is more likely to be associated with death than methicillin-sensitive *S. aureus* (MSSA) bacteremia (Table 2). A study of 504 bacteremia patients (316 MSSA, 188

TABLE 2 Studies Regarding the Effect of Methicillin Resistance and Outcomes in *Staphylococcus aureus* Bacteremia

Ref.	Study design	Total (*n*)	Patient group	Patients included MRSA	Patients included MSSA	Patient deaths (%) MRSA	Patient deaths (%) MSSA	OR/RR (95% CI)
Whitby et al. (2001) (8)	Meta-analysis of 9 studies	2208	All	778	1430	29	12	2.12 (1.76–2.57) (fixed effect method) 20.03 (1.55–2.65) (random effect method)
Cosgrove et al. (2003) (9)	Meta-analysis of 31 studies	3963	All	1360	2603	Not reported	Not reported	1.93 (1.54–2.42) (random effect model)
Blot et al. (2002) (10)	Cohort study + multivariate survival analysis 2 case-control studies	85	ICU	47	38	53	18	1.93 (1.18–3.18) (hazard ratio)

Talon et al. (2002) (11)	Cohort study, multivariate analysis	99	All	30	6	43.3	20.3	2.97 (1.12–7.88)
Melzer et al. (2003) (12)	Cohort study, logistic regression analysis	815	All	382	433	11.8	5.1	1.72 (0.92–3.20)
Kim et al. (2003) (13)	Cohort study, logistic regression analysis	238	All	127	111	40.2	33.3	In eradicable foci group ($n = 96$): 0.84 (1.24–2.97) In noneradicable foci group ($n = 142$): 2.40 (1.19–4.83)
Gastmeier et al. (2006) (14)	National cohort study, multivariable analysis	378	ICU	95	283	16.8	6.0	3.84 (1.51–10.2)

Abbreviations: MRSA, methicillin-resistant *S. aureus*; MSSA, methicillin-sensitive *S. aureus*; OR, odds ratio; RR, risk ratio.

MRSA) documented that the overall mortality rate was 22%, but MRSA bacteremia was associated with a 1.68-fold higher risk of death compared to MSSA patients (15).

MRSA bacteremia in ICU patients was associated with a 1.9-fold increased risk of in-hospital death compared to MSSA bacteremia patients (10). The impact of methicillin resistance on mortality was examined in a meta-analysis of nine studies, concluding that MRSA bacteremia was associated with a twofold increased risk of death (95% CI, 1.55–2.65) (8). A second meta-analysis of 31 cohort studies (1980–2000, $n = 3963$) determined that MRSA bacteremia was associated with an attributable mortality that was 2.16-fold higher compared with MSSA bacteremia (OR, 1.93) (9). Similarly, a study of 378 cases of *S. aureus* primary bacteremia in ICU patients documented a higher mortality rate in MRSA patients (16.8% vs. 6%) and only MRSA was significantly associated with death from *S. aureus* primary bacteremia (OR, 3.84; CI, 1.51–10.2) (14). Furthermore, community-dwelling, hemodialysis-dependent patients hospitalized with MRSA bacteremia face a higher mortality risk, longer hospital stay, and higher inpatient costs than patients with MSSA bacteremia (16).

MRSA bacteremia is also associated with increased resource utilization. In a study of hospital costs attributable to *S. aureus* bacteremia, it was found that MRSA had nearly twice the cost relative to MSSA ($21,577 vs. $11,668) (17). A study of 348 patients with *S. aureus* bacteremia (96 with MRSA) documented that MRSA bacteremia was associated with significantly increased duration of hospitalization (1.29-fold increase) and hospital charges (1.36-fold increase) (18).

CA-MRSA BACTEREMIA

CA-MRSA bacteremia is also on the rise. Compared with nosocomial MRSA strains, CA-MRSA strains are more susceptible to non-β-lactam antimicrobials (e.g., clindamycin), trimethoprim-sulfamethoxazole, and tetracyclines (e.g., doxycycline). CA-MRSA strains are also associated with greater toxin production compared with nosocomial MRSA strains. The distinction between nosocomial and CA-MRSA strains is becoming blurred. CA-MRSA strains are emerging as major causes of nosocomial infection. The USA300 strain was identified as the causative pathogen in 67% of invasive CA-MRSA infections and in 22% of nosocomial MRSA infections (19). The majority (65%) of bloodstream MRSA isolates were CA-MRSA strains in a recent study from Houston. Similarly, MRSA USA300 genotype, the predominant cause of CA-MRSA infections in the Atlanta area, has now emerged as a significant cause of health care–associated and nosocomial bloodstream infection (20). Mathematical modeling strongly suggests that CA-MRSA will become the dominant MRSA strain in hospitals and health care facilities in the near future (21,22).

DIAGNOSIS

The diagnosis of MRSA bacteremia is made by isolation of MRSA from blood cultures obtained in patients with presumed systemic infection. Nosocomial bacteremia is defined as a case of bacteremia arising two or more days after admission to hospital as recommended by the Centers for Disease Control and Prevention (23). Peripheral blood cultures should be utilized for determination of bacteremia whenever possible.

RISK FACTORS FOR MRSA BACTEREMIA

A number of risk factors for MRSA bacteremia have been identified, including male gender, admission due to trauma, immunosuppression, presence of a central venous catheter or an indwelling urinary catheter, and a past history of MRSA infection (7,24). Other variables associated with MRSA bacteremia include increased age, severe underlying disease (e.g., liver disease, diabetes, renal failure), neurologic disease, intravenous drug use, recent hospitalization, previous antibiotic therapy, and nursing home residence (25,26). Invasive procedures (e.g., catheterization, intubation, surgery) result in disruption of mucocutaneous barriers and are also risk factors. Some experts suggest that the best way to distinguish patients at risk for MRSA is to consider age, underlying medical conditions, previous antibiotic exposure, and the origin of the infection (hospital acquired, health care associated, or community acquired). The single most important predictor of MRSA bacteremia is recent prior antibiotic therapy. The presence of decubitus ulcers was also identified as an independent risk factor (27).

Independent risk factors that have been identified for ICU-acquired MRSA infections include the following:

- Hospitalization period in an ICU (OR, 1.090; 95% CI, 1.038–1.144; *p*, 0.001)
- Central venous catheter insertion (OR, 1.822; 95% CI, 1.095–3.033; *p*, 0.021)
- Previous antibiotic use (OR, 2.337; 95% CI, 1.326–4.119; *p*, 0.003)
- Presence of more than two patients having nasal colonization in the same ICU at the same time (OR, 1.398; 95% CI, 1.020–1.917; *p*, 0.037) (28)

MRSA colonization (either nares or wound) has been confirmed as an independent risk factor for subsequent MRSA infection in ICU patients (OR, 3.84; *p*, 0.0003) (29).

MANAGEMENT OF MRSA BACTEREMIA

Early diagnosis of bacteremia should be sought in order to implement adequate treatment, including prompt appropriate antimicrobial therapy. Inadequate antimicrobial therapy (defined as empiric antibiotic therapy including no antibiotic to which the isolate was susceptible) is a significant risk factor for mortality (30,31). In a study of 549 patients with

S. aureus sterile site infections, logistic regression analysis identified inappropriate initial antimicrobial treatment as an independent determinant (OR, 1.92) of hospital mortality (32). The importance of appropriate (i.e., anti-MRSA) initial empiric antibiotic therapy for patients at risk for MRSA bacteremia is clear. Delay in appropriate antibiotic therapy is also a risk factor for adverse outcome (33). A recent study documented that initial antibiotic therapy was inappropriate in 35% of cases of *S. aureus* bacteremia, and time to effective antibiotic therapy was longer in methicillin-resistant cases (25.5 vs. 9.6 hours; *p*, 0.0005) (34).

S. aureus bacteremia is associated with serious complications including endocarditis in 30% to 40% of cases (35,36). Blood cultures should be repeated three days following initiation of antistaphylococcal antibiotic therapy in all patients with *S. aureus* bacteremia. Patients with positive blood cultures at three days should undergo echocardiography to screen for the presence of endocarditis (Fig. 1). Factors predictive of endocarditis include underlying valvular heart disease, history of prior endocarditis, intravenous drug use, community acquisition of bacteremia, and an unrecognized source. Hematuria in the setting of staphylococcemia is an important clue to coexisting *S. aureus* infective endocarditis. Hematuria may arise by two mechanisms: renal infarction by embolization or immunologically mediated glomerulonephritis. Transesophageal echocardiography (TEE) can visualize much smaller vegetations and can better detect complications, such as valve perforation and abscesses. Therefore, TEE permits earlier detection and initiation of therapy for endocarditis.

ERADICABLE VS. NONERADICABLE FOCUS OF INFECTION

In addition to antimicrobial therapy, "source control" or "focus identification and eradication" of the MRSA infection is of paramount importance. Drainage of suppurative collections and removal of infected devices that are the source of the MRSA bacteremia are necessary.

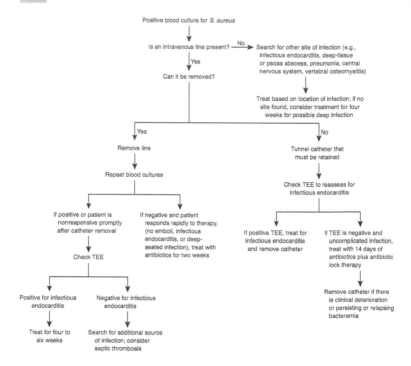

FIGURE 1 Management of *S. aureus* bacteremia. *Abbreviation*: TEE, transesophageal echocardiograpy. *Source*: From Ref. 37.

Eradicable foci of MRSA infection include surgically removable infections, drainable abscesses, and indwelling foreign bodies (implants, devices, and catheters). A large percentage (25% and higher) of patients with MRSA bacteremia are related to intravascular catheters, which are eradicable foci of infection. Infected intravascular catheters should be promptly removed and placed at a new site, and guidewire exchange of short-term intravascular catheters is contraindicated. Once an eradicable source has been addressed, systematic evaluation of the adequacy of source control must be undertaken. This can be accomplished through direct observation of wounds or radiographic evaluation such as ultrasound or CT scanning of deep infections. Noneradicable foci of MRSA infection include an infection of an unknown primary site, pneumonia, endocarditis, and osteomyelitis or arthritis. Noneradicable focus of infection is an independent predictor of mortality in *S. aureus* bacteremia (13).

ANTIBIOTIC TREATMENT OF MRSA AND MSSA BACTEREMIA

Penicillinase-resistant penicillins (methicillin, oxacillin, nafcillin, flucloxacillin) are the antimicrobial agents of choice for *S. aureus* bacteremia because of methicillin-sensitive strains. Vancomycin or first-generation cephalosporins are alternatives but have lower antimicrobial activity than methicillin.

Vancomycin therapy has long been the therapy of choice for MRSA bacteremia. Combination therapy with gentamicin may be useful for the first few days of treatment in selected patients, but there are few prospective randomized data to support the use of combination regimens in *S. aureus* bacteremia. Newer antimicrobial agents, including linezolid, daptomycin, and dalbavancin, also have documented efficacy in the treatment of MRSA bacteremia (Table 3).

Although a rise in CA-MRSA has been documented in skin and skin structure infections (38), the vast majority of bloodstream infections are related to health care–associated MRSA (39). Other antimicrobial agents that are being used for the treatment of CA-MRSA skin infections, such as trimethoprim/sulfamethoxazole, clindamycin, tetracyclines, and fluoroquinolones, should not be utilized in the treatment of MRSA bacteremia (40).

TABLE 3 Antibiotics Available for Treatment of MRSA Bacteremia

Antibiotic	Route	Dose	Advantages	Disadvantages
Vancomycin	IV	1 g IV q12h, titrated by weight and renal function, recommendations to achieve higher trough concentrations (15–20 µg/mL) in pneumonia	Familiarity	Poor clinical outcome
			Low cost	Increased vancomycin MICs
				Dosage adjustment and monitoring of levels required
Linezolid	IV or PO	600 mg IV q12h	No dosage adjustment in renal or hepatic failure	Thrombocytopenia
				Cost
Daptomycin	IV	6 mg/kg IV qD	Once-daily dosing	Emerging bacterial resistance
				Cost
Dalbavancin	IV	1000 mg IV followed by 500 mg IV 1 wk later	Once-weekly dosing	Lack of familiarity
				Cost

Abbreviations: IV, intravenously; MICs, minimum inhibitory concentrations.

Vancomycin

Vancomycin has long been the standard treatment for MRSA bacteremia
(41). Vancomycin has recently been associated with suboptimal clinical
outcomes. A number of reports have documented persistence of MRSA
bacteremia with vancomycin therapy (42,43). Interestingly, vancomycin
success in the treatment of MSSA bacteremia may also be problematic in
comparison to the semisynthetic penicillins. Initial vancomycin therapy
was also associated with a higher incidence of delayed clearance (3 days)
of MSSA bacteremia (56.3 vs. 37.0%; *p*, 0.03) (30).

Recent studies have identified a relationship between antimicrobial
treatment success with vancomycin and decreased vancomycin MICs
(0.5 mg/mL vs. 1.0–2.0 mg/mL; *p*, 0.02). Clinical cure rates in bacteremia
treatment with vancomycin were higher (55.6%) for patients with MRSA
isolates with vancomycin MICs 0.5 mg/mL whereas vancomycin was
only 9.5% effective in cases in which vancomycin MICs for MRSA were
higher (1–2 mg/mL). A significant risk for vancomycin treatment failure
in MRSA bacteremia begins to emerge with increasing vancomycin MICs
well within the susceptible range (44). Because of mounting clinical data
that suggest a poor response to vancomycin therapy for isolates with a
vancomycin MIC of 4 mg/mL, the Clinical and Laboratory Standards
Institute has recently lowered the intermediate breakpoint to include
vancomycin MICs of 4 mg/mL; MIC breakpoints for vancomycin and
staphylococci include the following: susceptible, 2 mg/mL; intermediate,
4 to 16 mg/mL; and resistance, 32 mg/mL (45).

In a recent survey of infectious disease consultants asked about
persistent bacteremia due to MRSA with a vancomycin MIC approaching
the limit of the susceptible range, most indicated that they would switch
to newer antimicrobial agents for treatment (46).

Adverse events related to vancomycin include red-man syndrome
if the drug is infused too rapidly, and risk for renal toxicity, particularly if
utilized with other nephrotoxic drugs such as the aminoglycosides.
Increased usage of vancomycin over the past 20 years has also correlated

with increased vancomycin-resistant enterococci (VRE), and VRE colonization is associated with increased risk for VRE infection.

Linezolid

Linezolid is a bacteriostatic oxazolidinone antibiotic that has been proven effective for the treatment of patients with pneumonia and complicated skin and skin structure infection. Some studies have documented that linezolid has statistically, significantly higher clinical cure rates compared to vancomycin for pneumonia (47) and complicated skin infections (48). Linezolid-resistant MRSA is rare, but does exist (49,50).

The randomized, open-label, multicenter trial of linezolid versus vancomycin for the treatment of resistant gram-positive infections in children enrolled 113 patients with bacteremia. Clinical cure rates were not different for bacteremia patients (84.8% linezolid vs. 80% vancomycin for catheter-related bacteremia; 79.2% linezolid vs. 69.2% vancomycin for bacteremia of unknown source) (51).

A pooled analysis of prospective randomized studies comparing linezolid to vancomycin identified 144 adults with *S. aureus* bacteremia. Of 99 clinically evaluable patients with *S. aureus* bacteremia, primary infection was cured in 55% of linezolid recipients compared to 52% of vancomycin recipients. Clinical cure in MRSA bacteremia patients was 56% for linezolid compared to 46% for vancomycin. No differences in microbiologic success or overall survival were identified between the two groups. In the multivariate analysis, the treatment group was not a significant predictor of clinical cure or survival (52).

A systematic review of the published evidence for linezolid use in treatment of patients with endocarditis suggested that linezolid may be considered as a therapeutic option in the treatment of endocarditis due to multidrug-resistant gram-positive cocci (53). A recently completed prospective study compared linezolid to vancomycin in catheter-related bacteremia, but these data are not yet published.

Adverse events related to linezolid include bone marrow suppression, particularly thrombocytopenia; however, the incidence was no different than that related to vancomycin use in the treatment of patients with pneumonia (54).

Daptomycin

Daptomycin is a cyclic lipopeptide antibiotic that is rapidly bactericidal in vitro against most clinically relevant gram-positive bacteria, including *S. aureus*. Daptomycin is approved by the FDA for treatment of complicated skin and skin structure infections at a dose of 4 mg/kg/day IV, and is now approved for the treatment of bacteremia and endocarditis.

An open-label randomized noninferiority trial compared daptomycin (6 mg/kg IV daily) with standard therapy (vancomycin 1 g IV q 12 hours with appropriate dose adjustment or antistaphylococcal penicillin; with gentamicin 1 mg/kg IV q 8 hours for first four days) in patients with *S. aureus* bacteremia with or without endocarditis (55). At the end of therapy, the success rates were 61.7% in the daptomycin group compared to 60.9% in the standard therapy group. There was no difference in the outcome at 42 days after the end of therapy between groups (44.2% daptomycin vs. 41.7% standard therapy, modified intention-to-treat group).

MRSA was isolated from 45 of 120 patients who were treated with daptomycin (37.5%) and 44 of 115 patients who were treated with standard therapy (38.3%). Success rates favored daptomycin over vancomycin among the MRSA cohort (44.4% daptomycin, 31.8% standard therapy, $p = 0.28$) but were higher among patients receiving standard therapy for MSSA infection (44.6% daptomycin, 48.6% standard therapy, $p = 0.74$). This study concluded that daptomycin is not inferior to standard therapy for *S. aureus* bacteremia and right-sided endocarditis.

A recent separate subset analysis of patients infected with MRSA isolates (56) documented that 20 of the 45 (44.4%) daptomycin patients and 14 of the 43 (32.6%) vancomycin/gentamicin patients were successfully treated (difference 11.9%; confidence interval: 8.3–32.1). Success rates for daptomycin versus vancomycin/gentamicin were 45% versus 27% in complicated bacteremia, 60% versus 45% in uncomplicated bacteremia, and 50% versus 50% in right-sided MRSA endocarditis. Cure rates in patients with septic emboli and in patients who received pre-enrolment vancomycin were similar between treatment groups. However, in both treatment groups, success rates were lower in the elderly ($\geq$75 years). Persisting or relapsing bacteremia occurred in 27% of daptomycin and 21% of vancomycin/gentamicin patients; among these patients, MICs of $\geq$2 mg/L occurred in five daptomycin and four vancomycin/gentamicin patients. The clinical course of several patients may have been influenced by lack of surgical intervention.

Importantly, 6 of 19 patients who received daptomycin and had microbiologic treatment failure (32%) were found to have isolates that had developed resistance to daptomycin (MIC 2 mg/mL). Therefore, if treatment with daptomycin appears to be associated with clinical or microbiologic failure (i.e., persistent fever, symptoms, bacteremia) in patients with bacteremia, the emergence of daptomycin resistance should be carefully assessed including repeat cultures with sensitivities. Interestingly, clinically significant renal dysfunction occurred in a significantly lower percentage of patients who received daptomycin compared to standard therapy (11.0% vs. 26.3%, $p = 0.0004$). Daptomycin use is associated with myopathy, and creatine kinase and myoglobin should be monitored on a weekly or biweekly basis for the duration of therapy.

Dalbavancin

Dalbavancin is a new, semisynthetic glycopeptide antibiotic with excellent activity against gram-positive bacteria. Dalbavancin has a long half-life (9–12 days), which is longer than that of any currently available glycopeptide. A phase II, open-label, randomized multicenter study has confirmed the efficacy and safety of weekly dalbavancin therapy for catheter-related bacteremia caused by gram-positive pathogens (57). This prospective trial compared dalbavancin given in two doses administered one week apart, compared with a 14-day course of twice-daily vancomycin in the treatment of adult patients ($n = 75$) with catheter-related bacteremia. The overall success rate for the primary efficacy population (microintention-to-treat group patients infected with a protocol-defined gram-positive pathogen at baseline who received one dose of study medication) for patients treated with dalbavancin was 87% compared with 50% for the vancomycin group. Dalbavancin was statistically superior to vancomycin therapy. Furthermore, both treatment arms were more successful if the catheter was removed than if it was retained at baseline. Full FDA approval for dalbavancin is pending further phase III trials.

COMBINATION THERAPY

While some data suggest superiority of combinations therapy in treatment of MSSA infections, there are little data in support of combination therapy in MRSA bacteremia. Combination therapy using daptomycin together with gentamicin, rifampin, or fusidic acid has shown some promise in vitro, but no clinical in vivo data exist to support this practice.

COMPLICATIONS RELATED TO MRSA BACTEREMIA

S. aureus bacteremia is associated with a high mortality rate and a high likelihood of life-threatening complications including infective endocarditis and metastatic infections (58). MRSA bacteremia may also lead to several complications including infective endocarditis, sepsis, or metastatic foci of infection. About 12% of patients with *S. aureus* bacteremia have infective endocarditis (12). Metastatic complications, including distant abscesses in bones, joints, and other sites related to hematogenous dissemination, have been reported in up to 50% of patients with *S. aureus* bacteremia (59,60). In addition, patients with prosthetic devices, such as orthopedic prosthesis or pacemakers, who develop *S. aureus* bloodstream infections are prone to seeding of those devices. Other complications of *S. aureus* infections such as Waterhouse-Friderichsen syndrome and Henoch–Schoenlien purpura also occur with MRSA bacteremia.

DURATION OF ANTIMICROBIAL THERAPY

The optimal duration of antibiotic treatment for *S. aureus* bacteremia remains unknown. Duration of antimicrobial therapy is dependent on the severity of infection, specifically whether the infection is complicated or uncomplicated. The recommended duration of antibiotic therapy for complicated MRSA bacteremia is four to six weeks based on clinical response to treatment (61). Uncomplicated bacteremia is defined as a catheter-associated infection with removal of the catheter followed by negative repeat blood cultures and defervescense within 72 hours. Furthermore, there must be no evidence of endocarditis by transesophageal echocardiogram, no prosthetic material in joints or the intravascular space, and no evidence of metastatic infection (36). These uncomplicated infections should be treated with antibiotics for 14 days. Some advocate for longer therapy citing other factors such as the presence of thrombosis in catheter-associated bacteremia as reasons why longer antibiotic therapy may be needed to clear bacteremia (62).

There is, however, a lack of data from prospective randomized clinical trials to guide our management. A prospective observational study of 278 patients with *S. aureus* bacteremia determined that a duration of 14 days for antimicrobial treatment was associated with lower mortality (4% vs. 23%) and logistic regression analysis confirmed both 14 days of antimicrobial therapy and focus of infection removal as independent factors associated with reduced mortality (63). Some studies have suggested that a shorter duration of antibiotic treatment is a possible risk factor for recurrence. A retrospective cohort study of 397 patients with *S. aureus* infection complicated by bacteremia documented no association between duration of therapy 14 days or less and recurrence. However, being HIV-infected, having diabetes, or having an infection due to MRSA (OR, 2.11) were independent risk factors for recurrence, and these patients require more careful follow-up (64). Patients with endocarditis require four to eight weeks of intravenous antibiotics with or without surgery.

PREVENTION

Prevention of MRSA bacteremia is the ideal strategy. Previous exposure to antibiotics is the strongest risk factor for MRSA bacteremia (27,39). Minimizing unnecessary exposure to antibiotics is therefore strongly recommended as a preventive strategy. All efforts to prevent catheter-related blood stream infections, including minimizing the use of central venous catheters, should be initiated as a preventive strategy since the presence of a central venous catheter is a significant risk factor for the development of *S. aureus* bacteremia (65). The NNIS system data documented that 87% of bloodstream infections were associated with central venous catheters. Routine hospital infection controls measures used to stem the spread of MRSA include screening and isolating or cohorting patients and attempts to improve compliance with handwashing and the use of gloves.

CONCLUSIONS

Nosocomial bacteremia is a life-threatening infection. Coagulase-negative staphylococci and MRSA are the two most common causative pathogens. Initial empiric antimicrobial therapy for nosocomial bacteremia should include anti-MRSA antibiotics and be administered in a timely manner. Concomitant eradication of the source of the infection, including removal of intravascular catheters if necessary, is an important component of effective therapy.

REFERENCES

1. Richards MJ, Edwards JR, Culver DH, et al. Nosocomial infections in medical intensive care units in the U.S. National Nosocomial Infections Surveillance System. Crit Care Med 1999; 27(5):887–892.
2. Richards MJ, Edwards JR, Culver DH, et al. Nosocomial infections in combined medical-surgical intensive care units in the United States. Infect Control Hosp Epidemiol 2000; 21(8):510–515.
3. Wisplinghoff H, Bischoff T, Tallent SM, et al. Nosocomial bloodstream infections in US hospitals: analysis of 24,719 cases from a prospective nationwide surveillance study. Clin Infect Dis 2004; 39:309.
4. Gaynes R, Edwards JR, National Nosocomial Infections Surveillance System. Overview of nosocomial infections caused by gram-negative bacilli. Clin Infect Dis 2005; 41(6):848–854.
5. NNIS System. National Nosocomial Infections Surveillance (NNIS) System report, data summary from January 1992 through June 2004, issued October 2004. Am J Infect Control 2004; 32:470–485.
6. Styers D, Sheehan DJ, Hogan P, et al. Laboratory-based surveillance of current antimicrobial resistance patterns and trends among *Staphylococcus aureus*: 2005 status in the United States. Ann Clin Microbiol Antimicrob 2006; 5:2.
7. Barrett FF, McGehee RF, Finland M. Methicillin resistant *Staphylococcus aureus* at Boston City Hostpital. N Engl J Med 1968; 279:441–448.
8. Whitby M, McLaws ML, Berry G. Risk of death from methicillin-resistant *Staphylococcus aureus* bacteremia: a meta-analysis. Med J Aust 2001; 175(5): 264–267.
9. Cosgrove SE, Sakoulas G, Perencevich EN, et al. Comparison of mortality associated with methicillin-resistant and methicillin-susceptible *Staphylococcus aureus* bacteremia: a meta-analysis. Clin Infect Dis 2003; 36(1):53–59.
10. Blot SI, Vandewoude KH, Hoste EA, et al. Outcome and attributable mortality in critically ill patients with bacteremia involving methicillin-susceptible and methicillin-resistant *Staphylococcus aureus*. Arch Intern Med 2002; 162: 2229–2235.

11. Talon D, Woronoff-Lemsi MC, Limat S, et al. The impact of resistance to methicillin in *Staphylococcus aureus* bacteremia on mortality. Eur J Intern Med 2002; 13:31–36.
12. Melzer M, Eykyn SJ, Gransden WR, et al. Is methicillin-resistant *Staphylococcus aureus* more virulent than methicillin-susceptible *S. aureus*? A comparative cohort study of British patients with nosocomial infect and bacteremia. Clin Infect Dis 2003; 37:1453–1460.
13. Kim SH, Park WB, Lee KD, et al. Outcome of *Staphylococcus aureus* bacteremia in patients with eradicable foci versus noneradicable foci. Clin Infect Dis 2003; 27:794–799.
14. Gastmeier P, Sohr D, Geffers C, et al. Mortality risk with nosocomial *Staphylococcus aureus* infections in intensive care units: results from the German Nosocomial Infection Surveillance System (KISS). Infection 2005; 33(2):50–55.
15. Selvey LA, Whitby M, Johnson B. Nosocomial methicillin-resistant *Staphylococcus aureus* bacteremia: is it any worse than nosocomial methicillin-sensitive *Staphylococcus aureus* bacteremia? Infect Control Hosp Epidemiol 2000; 21(10):645–648.
16. Reed SD, Friedman JY, Engemann JJ, et al. Costs and outcomes among hemodialysis-dependent patients with methicillin-resistant or methicillin-susceptible *Staphylococcus aureus* bacteremia. Infect Control Hosp Epidemiol 2005; 26(2):175–183.
17. Lodise TP, McKinnon PS. Clinical and economic impact of methicillin resistance in patients with *Staphylococcus aureus* bacteremia. Diagn Microbiol Infect Dis 2005; 52(2):113–122.
18. Cosgrove SE, Qi Y, Kaye KS, et al. The impact of methicillin resistance in *Staphylococcus aureus* bacteremia on patient outcomes: mortality, length of stay, and hospital charges. Infect Control Hosp Epidemiol 2005; 26(2):166–174.
19. Klevens RM, Morrison MA, Nadle J, et al. Invasive methicillin-resistant *Staphylococcus aureus* infections in the United States. JAMA 2007; 298:1763–1771.
20. Seybold U, Kourbatova EV, Johnson JG, et al. Emergency of community-associated MRSA USA 300 genotype as a major cause of healthcare-associated bloodstream infections. Clin Infect Dis 2006; 42(5):647–656.
21. D'Agato EM, Webb FT, Horn MA, et al. Modeling the invasion of community-acquired MRSA into hospitals. Clin Infect Dis 2009; 48(3):274–284.
22. Gonzalez BE, Rueda AM, Shelburne SA, et al. Community-associated strains of MRSA as the cause of healthcare-associated infection. Infect Control Hosp Epidemiol 2006; 27(10):1051–1056.

23. Garner JS, Jarvis WR, Emori TG, et al. CDC definitions for nosocomial infections. Am J Infect Control 1988; 16:128–140.
24. Yoshida T, Tsushima K, Tsuchiya A, et al. Risk factors for hospital-acquired bacteremia. Intern Med 2005; 44(11):1157–1162.
25. Lesens O, Hansmann Y, Brannigan E, et al. Healthcare-associated *Staphylococcus aureus* bacteremia and the risk for methicillin resistance: is the CDC definition for community-acquired bacteremia still appropriate? Infect Control Hosp Epidemiol 2005; 26:204–209.
26. Rezende NA, Blumberg HM, Metzger BS, et al. Risk factors for methicillin resistance among patients with *Staphylococcus aureus* bacteremia at the time of hospital admission. Am J Med Sci 2002; 323(3):117–123.
27. Lodise TP Jr., McKinnon PS, Rybak M. Prediction model to identify patients with *Staphylococcus aureus* bacteremia at risk for methicillin resistance. Infect Control Hosp Epidemiol 2003; 24(9):655–661.
28. Oztoprak N, Cevik MA, Akinci E, et al. Risk factors for ICU-acquired methicillin-resistant *Staphylococcus aureus* infections. Am J Infect Control 2006; 34(1):1–5.
29. Garrouste-Orgeas M, Timsit JF, Kallel H, et al. Colonization with methicillin-resistant *Staphylococcus aureus* in ICU patients: morbidity, mortality, and glycopeptide use. Infect Control Hosp Epidemiol 2001; 22(11):687–692.
30. Guilarde AO, Turchi MD, Martelli CM, et al. *Staphylococcus aureus* bacteremia: incidence; risk factors and predictors for death in a Brazilian teaching hospital. J Hosp Infect 2006; 63(3):330–336.
31. Ibrahim EH, Sherman G, Ward S, et al. The influence of inadequate antimicrobial treatment of bloodstream infections on patient outcomes in the ICU. Chest 2000; 118(1):146–155.
32. Schramm GE, Johnson JA, Doherty JA, et al. Methicillin-resistant *Staphylococcus aureus* sterile-site infection: the importance of appropriate initial antimicrobial treatment. Crit Care Med; 34(8):2069–2074.
33. Lodise TP, McKinnon PS, Swiderski L, et al. Outcomes analysis of delayed antibiotic treatment for hospital-acquired *Staphylococcus aureus* bacteremia. Clin Infect Dis 2003; 36(11):1418–1423.
34. Khatib R, Saeed S, Sharma M, et al. Impact of initial antibiotic choice and delayed appropriate treatment on the outcome of *Staphylococcus aureus* bacteremia. Eur J Clin Microbiol Infect Dis 2006; 25(3):181–185.
35. Chang FY, MacDonald BB, Peacock JE Jr., et al. A prospective multicenter study of *Staphylococcus aureus* bacteremia: incidence of endocarditis, risk

factors for mortality, and clinical impact of methicillin resistance. Medicine 2003; 82:322–332.

36. Fowler VG Jr., Olsen MK, Corey GR, et al. Clinical identifiers of complicated *Staphylococcus aureus* bacteremia. Arch Intern Med 2003; 163:2066–2072.

37. Bamberger DM, Boyd SE. Management of *S. aureus* bacteremia. Am Fam Physician 2005; 72:2474–2481.

38. Moran GJ, Krishnadasan A, Gorwitz RJ, et al. EMERGEncy ID Net Study Group. Methicillin-resistant *S. aureus* infections among patients in the emergency department. N Engl J Med 2006; 355(7):666–674.

39. Naimi TS, LeDell KH, Como-Sabetti K, et al. Comparison of community- and health care-associated methicillin-resistant *Staphylococcus aureus* infection. JAMA 2003; 290(22):2976–2984.

40. Sabol KE, Echevarria KL, Lewis JS. Community-associated methicillin-resistant *Staphylococcus aureus*: new bug, old drugs. Ann Pharmacother 2006; 40:1125–1133.

41. Markowitz N, Quinn EL, Saravolatz LD. Trimethoprim-sulfamethoxazole compared with vancomycin for the treatment of *Staphylococcus aureus* infection. Ann Intern Med 1992; 117(5):390–398.

42. Khatib R, Riederer KM, Held M, et al. Protracted and recurrent MRSA bacteremia despite defervescence with vancomycin therapy. Scand J Infect Dis 1995; 27(5):529–532.

43. Fowler VG Jr, Sakoulas G, McIntyre LM, et al. Persistent bacteremia due to methicillin-resistant *Staphylococcus aureus* infection is associated with agr dysfunction and low-level in vitro resistance to thrombin induced platelet microbicidal protein. J Infect Dis 2004; 190:1140–1149.

44. Sakoulas G, Moise-Broder PA, Schentag J, et al. Relationship of MIC and bactericidal activity to efficacy of vancomycin for treatment of methicillin-resistant *Staphylococcus aureus* bacteremia. J Clin Microbiol 2004; 42(6): 2398–2402.

45. NCCLS. Performance standards for antimicrobial susceptibility testing: 16th informational supplement. NCCLS Document M100-S15. Wayne, PA: NCCLS, 2006.

46. Hageman JC, Liedtke LA, Sunenshine RH, et al.; the Infectious Diseases Society of American Emerging Infections Network. Management of persistent bacteremia cause by methicillin-resistant *Staphylococcus aureus*: a survey of infectious diseases consultants. Clin Infect Dis 2006; 43: e42–e45.

47. Kollef MH, Rello J, Cammarata SK, et al. Clinical cure and survival in Gram-positive ventilator-associated pneumonia: retrospective analysis of two double-blind studies comparing linezolid with vancomycin. Intensive Care Med 2004; 30(3):388–394.

48. Weigelt J, Itani K, Stevens D, et al. Linezolid versus vancomycin in treatment of complicated skin and soft tissue infections. Antimicrob Agents Chemother 2005; 49(6):2260–2266.

49. Hancock RE. Mechanisms of action of newer antibiotics for gram-positive pathogens. Lancet Infect Dis 2005; 5:209–218.

50. Ross JE, AndereggTR, Sader HS, et al. Trends in linezolid susceptibility patterns in 2002: report from the worldwide Zyvox Annual Appraisal of Potency and Spectrum Program. Diagn Microbiol Infect Dis 2005; 52:53–58.

51. Kaplan SL, Deville JG, Yogev R, et al.; the Linezolid Pediatric Study Group. Linezolid versus vancomycin for treatment of resistant gram-positive infections in children. Pediatr Infect Dis J 2003; 22(8):877–885.

52. Shorr AF, Kunkel MJ, Kollef M. Linezolid versus vancomycin for *Staphylococcus aureus* bacteraemia: pooled analysis of randomized studies. J Antimicrob Chemother 2005; 56(5):923–929.

53. Falagas ME, Manta KG, Ntziora F, et al. Linezolid for the treatment of patients with endocarditis: a systematic review of the published evidence. J Antimicrob Chemother 2006; 58(2):273–280.

54. Nasraway SA, Shorr AF, Kuter DJ, et al. Linezolid does not increase the risk of thrombocytopenia in patients with nosocomial pneumonia: comparative analysis of linezolid and vancomycin use. Clin Infect Dis 2003; 37(12): 1609–1616.

55. Fowler VG Jr., Boucher HW, Corey GR, et al. for the *S. aureus* Endocarditis and Bacteremia Study Group. Daptomycin versus standard therapy for bacteremia and endocarditis caused by *Staphylococcus aureus*. N Engl J Med 2006; 355(7):653–665.

56. Rehm SJ, Boucher H, Levine D, et al. Daptomycin versus vancomycin plus gentamicin for treatment of bacteremia and endocarditis due to *Staphylococcus aureus*: subset analysis of patients infected with methicillin-resistant isolates. J Antimicrob Chemother 2008; 62(6):1413–1421.

57. Raad I, Darouiche R, Vazquez J, et al. Efficacy and safety of weekly dalbavancin therapy for catheter-related bloodstream infection caused by grampositive pathogens. Clin Infect Dis 2005; 40:374–380.

58. Naber CK. *Staphylococcus aureus* bacteremia: epidemiology, pathophysiology and management strategies. CID 2009; 48:231–237.

59. Ringberg H, Thoren A, Lilja B. Metastatic complications of *Staphylococcus aureus* septicemia. To seek is to find. Infection 2000; 28(3):132–136.
60. Gottlieb GS, Fowler VG Jr., Kong LK, et al. *Staphylococcus aureus* bacteremia in the surgical patient: a prospective analysis of 73 postoperative patients who developed *Staphylococcus aureus* bacteremia at a tertiary care facility. J Am Coll Surg 2000; 190(1):50–57.
61. Mitchell DH, Howden BP. Diagnosis and management of *Staphylococcus aureus* bacteraemia. Intern Med J 2005; 35(suppl 2):S17–S24.
62. Corey GR. *Staphylococcus aureus* bloodstream infections: definitions and treatment. Clin Inf Dis 2009; 48:S254–S259.
63. Jensen AG, Wachmann CH, Espersen F, et al. Treatment and outcome of *Staphylococcus aureus* bacteremia: a prospective study of 278 cases. Arch Intern Med 2002; 162:25–32.
64. Kreisel K, Boyd K, Langenberg P, et al. Risk factors for recurrence in patients with *Staphylococcus aureus* infections complicated by bacteremia. Diagn Microbiol Infect Dis 2006; 55(3):179–184.
65. Jensen AG, Wachmann CH, Poulsen KB, et al. Risk factors for hospital-acquired *Staphylococcus aureus* bacteremia. Arch Intern Med 1999; 159:1437.

Antibiotics for MRSA Infections in the United States

R. Lawrence Reed
Department of Surgery, Loyola University Medical Center, Maywood, Illinois, U.S.A.

INTRODUCTION

Methicillin-resistant *Staphylococcus aureus* (MRSA) is a multidrug resistant organism. Depending on the MRSA strain, antibiotic resistance patterns have varied. All MRSA strains are, by definition, resistant to methicillin and other β-lactam antibiotics. However, resistance to other antimicrobials is common, especially in the case of health care–associated MRSA (HA-MRSA or USA100), which is usually resistant to aminoglycosides and fluoroquinolones in addition to β-lactam antibiotics.

Despite MRSA's resistance to several antimicrobials, there is a growing list of new agents that are effective against the organism. In addition, community-acquired MRSA (CA-MRSA, or USA300) is often sensitive to many traditional antibiotics, including minocycline, doxycycline, trimethoprim/sulfamethoxazole, rifampin, and clindamycin. HA-MRSA may occasionally be sensitive to these agents, but other agents are usually necessary to insure effective therapy.

The rising incidence of MRSA infections has actually produced a market opportunity for the development of new anti-MRSA antibiotics. Currently, there are four FDA-approved antibiotics for the treatment of MRSA infections: vancomycin, linezolid, daptomycin, and tigecycline (Table 1). Knowledge of the risks and benefits associated with each of these agents makes the clinician better able to optimize his patient's care.

TABLE 1 Antibiotics Having FDA Approval for Use in MRSA Infections

Drug	Approved indications (MRSA infections)	Routes of administration	Dosing	Comments
Vancomycin	Serious or severe infections (endocarditis, septicemia, bone infections, lower respiratory tract infections, skin and skin structure infections (1).	Intravenous (orally for *C. difficile* enterocolitis	1 g every 12 hrs	Poor tissue penetration; not as effective against MSSA as β-lactam agents
Linezolid	cSSTI, pneumonia	Intravenous or orally	600 mg twice daily	Oral bioavailability; excellent tissue penetration; evidence of superiority vs. vancomycin for MRSA pneumonia (2, 3), SSTI (4), and SSI (5); evidence of overall reduced costs of treatment, shorter hospital lengths of stay, fewer IV days (4, 6, 7) Higher acquisition costs than vancomycin often provokes restrictions to use

TABLE 1 Antibiotics Having FDA Approval for Use in MRSA Infections (*Continued*)

Drug	Approved indications (MRSA infections)	Routes of administration	Dosing	Comments
Daptomycin	cSSTI, bacteremia (including right-heart endocarditis)	Intravenous only	For cSSTI: 4 mg/kg daily For bacteremia: 6 mg/kg	Appears to cover MSSA as well as β-lactam agents and MRSA as well as vancomycin. May be associated with increased incidence of myopathy. Is inactivated by pulmonary surfactant, leading to inferior outcomes for treatment of pneumonia
Tigecycline	cSSTI, complicated intra-abdominal infections, community-acquired pneumonia	Intravenous only	100 mg initially, then 50 mg every 12 hr	Very broad spectrum of action. Very high (25–30%) incidence of nausea and vomiting

Abbreviations: MRSA, methicillin-resistant *Staphylococcus aureus*; MSSA, methicillin-sensitive *S. aureus*; cSSTI, complicated skin and soft tissue infection.

VANCOMYCIN

Vancomycin was first discovered in 1956 in some soil samples from Southeast Asia, where it was produced by an actinomycete, *Streptococcus orientalis* (8). Because of the previous emergence and prevalence of a penicillin-resistant *S. aureus* at the time, approval of the drug was fast-tracked by the FDA. It was first used clinically in 1958, a mere two years after it had been discovered (8). Early vancomycin preparations were problematic, with significant toxicity. Shortly after vancomycin's introduction, however, staphylococcus-resistant penicillins (such as methicillin and oxacillin) and the cephalosporins were developed, which were also effective against the penicillin-resistant *S. aureus*. Because of these developments and vancomycin's toxicity, subsequent use of vancomycin was sparse during its first two decades of clinical use. In the 1970s, the emergence of *Clostridium difficile* infections produced a new indication for vancomycin. Shortly thereafter, the rising incidence of MRSA, likely because of heavy β-lactam pressure from extended spectrum penicillins and cephalosporins, caused vancomycin use to escalate to alarming levels.

Vancomycin is a glycopeptide antimicrobial. It binds to the C-terminal end of late peptidoglycan precursors, preventing the effective formation of a bacterial cell wall (9). Its actions against bacteria are carried out on the outer surface of the bacterial cell membrane, as it cannot penetrate into the cytoplasm. Thus, vancomycin depends on the bacterial translocation of the cell wall precursors onto the outer surface of the microbial membrane.

Because vancomycin is effective against cell wall synthesis, it is active only against gram-positive organisms. Gram-positive organisms stain as they do because of the presence of the peptidoglycan cell wall. Gram-negative organisms do not have such a cell wall and are thus unaffected by vancomycin. Vancomycin is indicated for multiple infections because of gram-positive infections, including endocarditis, septicemia, bone infections, pneumonia, and skin and skin structure infections.

Vancomycin is administered intravenously for most infections, except in the occasional management of *C. difficile* enterocolitis, in which it is administered orally. Vancomycin is not absorbed from the oral route, although there have been cases of toxic levels being achieved after oral administration in patients who have had severe mucosal damage of the intestinal tract (10–13). Its apparent volume of distribution approximates total body water (10).

Rapid administration of vancomycin produces an abrupt histamine-like reaction commonly called the "red man syndrome." Administering the agent over a one-hour infusion time significantly reduces the incidence of this problem. Other idiosyncratic reactions can occur, however, including rashes. While the early vancomycin preparations were quite toxic, the current formulation is much safer. However, data suggest that administration of the combination of vancomycin and aminoglycoside antibiotics is more nephrotoxic (35%) than either agent alone (7%) (11).

There is increasing evidence that vancomycin may not achieve clinical results equivalent to its microbiological susceptibility. Clinical failure rates of >40% in the treatment of pneumonia have been demonstrated using standard dosing (12–14), MRSA bacteremia in vancomycin-treated patients may persist after defervescence and lead to delayed complications (15).

One study that illuminates vancomycin's shortcoming is that conducted by Gonzalez et al., evaluating 32 cases of MRSA and 54 cases of methicillin-sensitive *S. aureus* (MSSA) as etiologies of bacteremic pneumonia. Ten of 20 patients (50%) with MRSA pneumonia treated with vancomycin died. Of the cases with MSSA, 47% (8/17) treated with vancomycin died while none (0/10) treated with cloxacillin died. Thus, vancomycin did equally poorly against both MRSA and MSSA (16). Given the significantly better outcome with cloxacillin, the only rationale for vancomycin use is the presence of methicillin resistance. However, this study serves to make it increasingly obvious that vancomycin has some serious shortcomings with respect to its effectiveness.

The ability of standard doses of vancomycin to clear infection has been related to its plasma levels. Hyatt et al. demonstrated that patients with vancomycin concentrations having an area under the inhibitory curve (AUIC) of >125 had a 97% clinical success rate versus 50% for those with an AUIC <125 (17). Similarly, Moise et al. demonstrated that patients with an AUIC >345 had a 78% clinical success rate versus that of 24% for an AUIC of <346 (12).

In 2004, Sakoulas et al. reported on 30 patients with MRSA bacteremia in whom multivariate analysis revealed clinical success to be highly correlated with reduced vancomycin MICs (OR 35.46, $p = 0.020$). Patients with an MIC of ≤ 0.5 µg/mL had a 55.6% clinical success when treated with vancomycin whereas those with MICs in the 1.0 to 2.0 µg/mL range (still considered microbiologically sensitive) only had a 9.5% clinical success rate in response to vancomycin therapy (18). In 2008, Lodise and colleagues conducted a retrospective evaluation of 92 adult patients treated with vancomycin for MRSA bacteremia. Cases in which the vancomycin MIC was ≥ 1.5 mg/L were associated with a treatment failure rate over twice as high as those in which the vancomycin MIC was ≤ 1.0 mg/L (36.4% vs. 15.4%, $p = 0.049$). In addition, a Poisson regression analysis revealed that "a vancomycin MIC of >1.5 mg/liter was independently associated with failure (adjusted risk ratio, 2.6; 95% confidence interval, 1.3 to 5.4; $p = 0.01$)" (19).

In 2006, the Clinical Laboratory Standards Institute (CLSI) had dropped its sensitivity ranges for *S. aureus* to vancomycin to ≤ 2 µg/mL for vancomycin-sensitive *S. aureus* (VSSA), 4 to 8 µg/mL for vancomycin intermediate-sensitive strains (VISA), and ≥ 16 µg/mL for vancomycin-resistant strains (VRSA) (20). The Food and Drug Administration (FDA) followed suit in 2009, dropping to the same susceptibility ranges as the CLSI had set from the previously long-held ranges of ≤ 4 µg/mL, 8 to 16 µg/mL, and ≥ 32 µg/mL for VSSA, VISA, and VRSA (21,22).

The most apparent reason leading to these adjustments of clinical susceptibility breakpoints is the impaired ability of vancomycin to achieve tissue concentrations above the MIC. Cruciani determined that vancomycin frequently failed to maintain concentrations in human lung tissue that exceeded the MIC for susceptible staphylococci (23). Similar studies in heart valves, subcutaneous tissue, and muscle have demonstrated barely adequate vancomycin levels (24). Thus, it is eminently possible that vancomycin can demonstrate excellent in vitro effectiveness at relatively low concentrations in culture media but poor clinical (in vivo) effectiveness because those same concentrations cannot be achieved in tissue.

In recognition of this problem, it has been argued that raising trough level (≥ 15 µg/mL) could improve clinical results with vancomycin use (25). However, there are no prospective, randomized controlled clinical trials indicating that vancomycin efficacy is improved with such a practice, nor can we be assured that vancomycin toxicity will be avoided. In fact, there are recent studies that indicate that higher vancomycin trough levels do not improve clinical outcomes (19,26,27).

In addition to inadequate tissue level concentrations, another concern now affecting vancomycin use is the evidence of growing resistance to the drug. After vancomycin's introduction in the late 1950s, initial bacterial resistance to vancomycin was rare, primarily because of the scant use of the drug. With the emergence of MRSA, vancomycin became more heavily used as it was initially the only agent available for MRSA infections. The resulting increased use (and, often, overuse) of vancomycin has applied more antibiotic pressure toward the development of resistance. Vancomycin-resistant *Enterococcus* (VRE) began to emerge in the late 1980s, VISA emerged in the late 1990s, and VRSA began to emerge in the early 2000s. It appears that staphylococcal resistance to vancomycin has been acquired by transfer of a vanA gene from a VRE isolate rather than de novo mutation within the *S. aureus* species (28,29).

Attempts to improve vancomycin's effectiveness have combined it with rifampin (30) or aminoglycosides, although, again, there are no prospective data to confirm the validity of this practice. Continuous infusions of vancomycin may offer some advantages over intermittent twice-daily dosing, although such regimens are not considered standard at this time. However, in a prospective, randomized, multicenter trial, Wysocki et al. demonstrated that continuous vancomycin infusion was associated with lower administration costs, more rapid achievement of target concentrations, fewer monitoring samples, and reduced dosing variability in comparison to standard intermittent dosing (31).

LINEZOLID

Linezolid is the first of a new antibiotic class, the oxazolidinones. It was developed in the 1990s as a response to the rising incidence of MRSA and the increased use and emerging resistance to vancomycin. It was approved for clinical use by the FDA in April 2000. Its mechanism of action involves binding selectively to the bacterial 50S ribosomal subunit, where it inhibits the formation of a functional initiation complex. Linezolid is effective against gram-positive pathogens, such as *Enterococcus faecium*, *S. aureus*, *Streptococcus agalactiae*, *Strep. pneumoniae*, and *Strep. pyogenes*. It has almost no effect on gram-negative bacteria.

Unique among the anti-MRSA antibiotics is the 100% bioavailability of linezolid. An oral dose of 600 mg of linezolid achieves the same plasma concentrations as intravenously administered drug. In addition, tissue penetration is generally better than that of many other antibiotics, especially vancomycin. Plasma and epithelial lining fluid (ELF) concentrations of linezolid in healthy volunteers exceeded the minimum concentration need to inhibit 90% of organisms (MIC90) values for enterococci, staphylococci, and streptococci throughout the entire dosing interval (32). Indeed, it appears that linezolid is concentrated in lung tissue (similar to what has been observed for fluoroquinolones) in that ELF concentrations of linezolid exceed plasma concentrations by a mean of 206% ($\pm$26%) (33,34). Linezolid concentrations in skin blister fluid approach 104% of plasma concentrations (35).

Linezolid has acquired FDA approval for the treatment of the following: VRE infections, including cases with concurrent bacteremia; nosocomial pneumonia caused by *S. aureus* (MRSA and MSSA) or *Strep. pneumoniae* (including multidrug-resistant strains); complicated skin and skin structure infections, including diabetic foot infections, without concomitant osteomyelitis, because of MRSA, MSSA, *Strep. pyogenes*, or *Strep. agalactiae* (36). Linezolid is not indicated for catheter-related bloodstream infections or for infections due to gram-negative organisms.

Linezolid is generally well tolerated. However, there are some adverse effects that have received attention. A reversible myelosuppression (including anemia, leukopenia, pancytopenia, and thrombocytopenia) has been reported in patients receiving linezolid, typically in patients taking the drug for prolonged durations. This has prompted the recommendation that weekly monitoring of complete blood counts be performed in patients taking the drug for more than two weeks. Linezolid has the potential for interaction with adrenergic and serotonergic agents, as it is a reversible, nonselective inhibitor of monoamine oxidase. However, a review of 15 phase III and IV comparator-controlled clinical trials showed no evidence of an increased incidence of signs and symptoms of serotonin syndrome in patients treated concomitantly with linezolid and a selective serotonin reuptake inhibitor (37). Other side effects include rashes, loss of appetite, diarrhea, nausea, constipation, and fever. A few patients have experienced severe allergic reactions, tinnitus, and pseudomembranous colitis. Linezolid is a weak monoamine oxidase inhibitor and cannot be used with tyramine-containing foods or pseudoephedrine. Presumably because of linezolid's effect on bacterial ribosomes and the similarity to mitochondrial ribosomes, linezolid may be toxic to mitochondria, producing lactic acidosis and peripheral neuropathy in some patients (38). Peripheral neuropathy and optic neuropathy are rarely reported complications (39).

Although its clinical history is relatively brief, resistance to linezolid has already been reported, although rare. Because most bacteria have multiple copies of the 23S rRNA of the 50S ribosomal subunit to which linezolid binds, resistance requires multiple mutations of those copies of the 23S rRNA. However, staphylococcal resistance to linezolid has also been reported in human isolates because of a transferable rRNA methyltransferase gene, named *cfr* (40). Resistance to linezolid was initially reported for VRE isolates, but subsequently observed for *S. aureus,* typically following prolonged courses of linezolid (41). The highest linezolid resistance rate reported thus far is 4% for VRE isolates (42).

Linezolid has been proven effective for the treatment of complicated skin and soft-tissue infections (including diabetic foot infections) and for the treatment of pneumonia because of susceptible gram-positive organisms, including MRSA. An interesting set of studies combined the FDA registration studies for the pneumonia indication to determine if the resulting larger number of study patients could demonstrate against any superiority of linezolid compared to vancomycin. These reports demonstrated improved clinical cure rates and even survival rates for patients who received linezolid for the treatment of MRSA pneumonia (both hospital acquired and ventilator associated) than for those treated with vancomycin. Indeed, linezolid therapy fell out as an independent predictor of improved cure and survival (2,3). Similar suggestions of superiority over vancomycin have been demonstrated for linezolid treatment of MRSA skin and soft-tissue infections, including surgical site infections (5,43). The potential improved outcomes using linezolid compared to vancomycin, if true, could be attributed to the improved tissue penetration of linezolid previously discussed. Other clinical experience with linezolid has demonstrated a marked reduction in the hospital length of stay for the treatment of skin and soft-tissue infection as well as a reduced number of IV days (6,7,43,44). These studies have led to analyses indicating a significant health care cost savings despite the higher acquisition cost of linezolid.

DAPTOMYCIN

Daptomycin is a lipopeptide antibiotic active only against gram-positive organisms. It is a naturally occurring compound that is found in the soil saprotroph, *Streptomyces roseosporus*. Daptomycin binds to bacterial cell membranes in a concentration-dependent and calcium-requiring process, causing rapid depolarization. This results in a rapid bacterial cell death without cell lysis.

Daptomycin has proven in vitro activity against enterococci (including glycopeptide-resistant enterococci), staphylococci (including MRSA), streptococci, and corynebacteria. It was approved for use in skin and skin structure infections caused by gram-positive infections in September of 2003. In those studies, it was shown to have equivalent outcomes to approved comparator agents (either vancomycin or a semisynthetic penicillin) (45). Daptomycin also received FDA approval and for the treatment of *S. aureus* bacteremia and right-sided *S. aureus* endocarditis in May of 2006 (46).

Daptomycin is contraindicated for the treatment of pneumonia. Despite potent bactericidal activity against *Strep. pneumoniae*, daptomycin (4 mg/kg every 24 hours) failed to achieve statistical noninferiority against the comparator, ceftriaxone (2 g every 24 hours). Clinical efficacy in the pneumonia trial was 79% for daptomycin and 87% for ceftriaxone (47). The primary explanation for daptomycin's ineffectiveness in treating pneumonia is that pulmonary surfactant inactivates daptomycin, resulting in inhibition of antibacterial activity (48).

Daptomycin is only available using the intravenous route. Its pharmacokinetics indicates a nearly linear elimination rate. The drug is 92% protein bound, providing a half-life of over eight hours. The drug is typically dosed on a once-daily basis at 4 mg/kg for skin and soft-tissue infections, while the dose is increased to 6 mg/kg once daily for *S. aureus* bacteremia or right-sided endocarditis.

While nausea and vomiting are the most common adverse events noted with the drug, their incidence has not been any different from that of the comparator drugs. The specific adverse event that has received most attention, however, is the potential for myalgias and muscle enzyme (i.e., CPK) elevations, although this has usually occurred in <3% of treated patients. Nevertheless, physicians are advised to be alert to the potential for myopathy and rhabdomyolysis during daptomycin therapy. The simultaneous use of daptomycin with statins may potential the tendency toward myopathy, leading to the manufacturer's recommendation that statins be discontinued while taking daptomycin.

Because of its unique mechanism of action, it has been hoped that daptomycin would be less susceptible to the development of bacterial resistance than other agents. However, resistance has been reported for VRE and *S. aureus* (49–51). In some cases, it appears that resistance is coincident with an increased thickening of the staphylococcal bacterial cell wall, similar to that seen with VISA (52). Microbiological evaluation of daptomycin resistance suggests that resistant organisms frequently lose much of their virulence (53).

TIGECYCLINE

Tigecycline is the first clinically available drug in a new class of antibiotics called the glycylcyclines, which are structurally similar to the tetracyclines in that they contain a central four-ring carbocyclic skeleton. Tigecycline has a substitution at the D-9 position that is believed to confer broad-spectrum activity. Tigecycline targets the bacterial ribosome and is a bacteriostatic agent.

Tigecycline has an extremely broad spectrum of activity, affecting aerobes, anaerobes, gram-positive bacteria (including MRSA), and gram-negative bacteria [including those possessing extended-spectrum β-lactamase (ESBL) plasmids]. However, it has no activity against *Pseudomonas* or *Proteus*.

Tigecycline has received FDA approval for the treatment of complicated skin and soft-tissue infections, complicated intra-abdominal infections, and community-acquired pneumonia (54). The drug is only available for intravenous infusion, given as an initial 100 mg loading dose followed by 50 mg every 12 hours thereafter. Dose adjustments are necessary for patients with liver disease, but no adjustment is necessary for patients with impaired renal excretion.

OTHER ANTIBIOTICS WITH ACTIVITY AGAINST MRSA

Several older antibiotics have variable activity against MRSA but do not actually carry FDA approval for the treatment of MRSA infections. Many of these drugs can be administered orally and are often very useful in the treatment of community-acquired MRSA. Trimethoprim/sulfamethoxazole is often very effective against MRSA microbiologically (55), although in clinical studies it does not perform as well as vancomycin against MRSA (56). Long-acting tetracyclines such as minocycline and doxycycline have also demonstrated effectiveness against MRSA (57). Clindamycin is orally available and often effective against MRSA, although it occasionally develops an erythromycin-induced resistance, identified in the microbiology laboratory by the so-called "D test" (58). Other older agents that are occasionally useful in managing MRSA infections include rifampin, macrolides (i.e., clarithromycin), tetracycline, fluoroquinolones (moxifloxacin and levofloxacin), gentamicin, and chloramphenicol.

There are also newer antibiotics for MRSA infections whose FDA approval is pending. Three are lipoglycopeptides (as is vancomycin), two are cephalosporins, and one is a dihydrofolate reductase (DHFR) inhibitor (similar to trimethoprim).

Dalbavancin

Dalbavancin, a second-generation lipoglycopeptide agent belonging to the same class as vancomycin, is remarkable for an extremely long half-life that will allow for once-weekly intravenous dosing (59). A skin and soft-tissue infection study comparing dalbavancin with linezolid showed equivalent results with 90% of patients in both groups having a successful outcome (60).

Telavancin

Telavancin has entered the FDA approval process. It is a bactericidal lipoglycopeptide that has multiple mechanisms of action, including the inhibition of cell wall production via inhibition of transglycosylase activity as well as concentration-dependent cell membrane disruption.

Thus far, telavancin has been studied for the treatment of gram-positive complicated skin and soft-tissue infections. Two phase II studies compared treatment with telavancin to standard therapy (defined as either a semisynthetic penicillin or vancomyin). In the first study, patients with *S. aureus* infections treated with telavancin had an 80% cure rate versus 77% for standard therapy. In the case of patients infected with MRSA, 82% of the telavancin patients were cured versus 69% of the standard therapy group (61). The second phase II study was similarly designed, and had similar results; in patients infected with *S. aureus*, 96% of the telavancin patients were cured versus 90% of the standard therapy patients, with identical clinical cure rates for both groups in those patients infected with MRSA (62). Two parallel, randomized, double-blind, active-control, phase III studies of telavancin versus vancomycin for the treatment of complicated skin and skin structure infections have also been reported. These studies were combined, as they had a prespecified pooled analysis design. Cure rates for patients with MRSA infection were 91% for telavancin and 86% for vancomycin.

Oritavancin

Oritavancin is a semisynthetic glycopeptide in development for the treatment of gram-positive infections. It displays rapid concentration-dependent killing against MRSA, MSSA, and VRSA within one hour, against VSE within 11 to 24 hours, and VRE within 10 hours (63).

Among its advantages are its multiple mechanisms of action and its long half-life (64).

There have been two completed phase III and one phase II trials of oritavancin in the treatment of skin and soft-tissue infections, although the results are yet unpublished. There have also been two phase II trials for the treatment of bacteremia. In all of these studies, oritavancin demonstrated noninferiority to the comparator agents (vancomycin followed by oral cephalexin) (65).

Ceftobiprole

Ceftobiprole is a cephalosporin that has been engineered to have activity against many gram-positive organisms including MRSA (66,67). Ceftobiprole is a broad-spectrum pyrrolidinone cephen, which is β-lactamase stable and has a strong affinity for the penicillin-binding proteins PBP2α and PBP2χ (68,69). The importance of this mechanism is that the resistance of MRSA to β-lactams is mediated by PBP2α, which functions after the normal PBPs have been inactivated by β-lactams. Ceftobiprole forms a stable acyl-enzyme complex at the active site of PBP2α, creating a very stable inhibition of the enzyme and providing efficacy against MRSA.

Ceftobiprole is bactericidal and has activity against MRSA, VISA, and VRSA (70–73), as well as methicillin-resistant *S. epidermidis* (MRSE). Gram-negative activity appears to be similar to cefepime including pseudomonas, although activity against ESBL organisms is not present. Anaerobic activity is present for common gram-positive isolates from diabetic foot infections (74).

Safety date from phase I and phase II trials are encouraging and raise no serious toxicity questions (75). The drug is cleared by the kidneys and is dosed intravenously at 500 mg every 12 hours. No oral formation is available. Dosing for pseudomonas coverage is recommended at 500 mg every eight hours.

Two phase III trials of complicated skin and skin structure infections have been performed comparing ceftobiprole to vancomycin with prospective, randomized, double-blind, multi-institutional trial; ceftobiprole cured 93.3% of the clinically evaluable patients while vancomycin cured 93.3%, whereas in those patients infected with MRSA, ceftobiprole cured 91.8% and vancomycin cured 90.0% (76).

Ceftobiprole has also been studied for the treatment of community-acquired pneumonia in comparison to ceftriaxone with or without linezolid. In the clinically evaluable population with moderate to severe disease, ceftobiprole exhibited a clinical cure rate of 87% versus 88% for the comparator (77).

Ceftaroline

Ceftaroline is a broad-spectrum cephalosporin possessing broad-spectrum, time-depending bactericidal activity against multidrug-resistant gram-positive organisms, including MRSA, VISA, and MRSE, as well as a variety of enteric gram-negative organisms and some gram-positive anaerobes. It is the bioactive metabolite of ceftaroline fosamil, a cephalosporin prodrug.

Ceftaroline has been studied in a phase II clinical trial of complicated skin and skin structure infections. In comparison to vancomycin with or without aztreonam, ceftaroline demonstrated a clinical cure rate of 96.7% among clinically evaluable patients compared to 88.9% for the comparator regimen. It exhibited a favorable safety and tolerability profile, consistent with most cephalosporins (78).

Iclaprim

Iclaprim is a selective DHFR inhibitor, similar to trimethoprim. It preferentially prevents the synthesis of bacterial DNA and RNA (79). Iclaprim is able to inhibit bacterial DHFRs with little or no human enzyme inhibition at concentrations much higher than that needed for bacterial DHFR inhibition (79,80). It is rapidly bactericidal with a post-antibiotic effect lasting several hours. Iclaprim is active against *S. aureus*, including MRSA, VISA, and VRSA (80,81).

Similar to linezolid, iclaprim offers the potential for oral admin-istration. An oral formulation of iclaprim demonstrates ∼40% bioavail-ability (82). A phase II clinical study employing an "IV-to-oral" switch regimen was completed in December 2008 (82).

Two phase III clinical studies of complicated skin and skin struc-ture infections demonstrated that iclaprim 0.8 mg/kg every 12 hours was noninferior to linezolid (83).

SUMMARY

While infections because of MRSA continue to be problematic, it is reassuring that there is a growing list of effective antimicrobials that clinicians can use to treat the patients. Traditional vancomycin is often effective, but appears to be developing some problems with consistent effectiveness. Vancomycin is not ideal as an empiric antibiotic for gram-positive infections, as it does not cover MSSA as well as β-lactam antimicrobials. One notable feature of many of the newer agents is that in contrast to vancomycin, they cover MSSA as well as β-lactam agents while covering MRSA as well as vancomycin. Thus, more consistently, effective initial presumptive therapy can be initiated with these agents, with de-escalation to either vancomycin or a β-lactam based on subse-quent culture results.

REFERENCES

1. Vancomycin indications and usage. RxList Inc, 2006. Available at: http://www. rxlist.com/cgi/generic2/vancomycin_ids.htm. Accessed August 12, 2006.
2. Wunderink RG, Rello J, Cammarata SK, et al. Linezolid vs vancomycin: analysis of two double-blind studies of patients with methicillin-resistant *Staphylococcus aureus* nosocomial pneumonia. Chest 2003; 124:1789–1797.

3. Kollef MH, Rello J, Cammarata SK, et al. Clinical cure and survival in Gram-positive ventilator-associated pneumonia: retrospective analysis of two double-blind studies comparing linezolid with vancomycin. Intensive Care Med 2004; 30:388–394.

4. Weigelt J, Itani K, Stevens D, et al. Linezolid versus vancomycin in treatment of complicated skin and soft tissue infections. Antimicrob Agents Chemother 2005; 49:2260–2266.

5. Weigelt J, Kaafarani HM, Itani KM, et al. Linezolid eradicates MRSA better than vancomycin from surgical-site infections. Am J Surg 2004; 188:760–766.

6. Li JZ, Willke RJ, Rittenhouse BE, et al. Effect of linezolid versus vancomycin on length of hospital stay in patients with complicated skin and soft tissue infections caused by known or suspected methicillin-resistant staphylococci: results from a randomized clinical trial. Surg Infect (Larchmt) 2003; 4:57–70.

7. Li Z, Willke RJ, Pinto LA, et al. Comparison of length of hospital stay for patients with known or suspected methicillin-resistant *Staphylococcus* species infections treated with linezolid or vancomycin: a randomized, multicenter trial. Pharmacotherapy 2001; 21:263–274.

8. Anderson R, Higgins HJ, Pettinga C. Symposium: how a drug is born. Cincinnati J Med 1961; 42:49–60.

9. Courvalin P. Vancomycin resistance in gram-positive cocci. Clin Infect Dis 2006; 42(suppl 1):S25–S34.

10. Reed RL II, Wu AH, Miller-Crotchett P, et al. Pharmacokinetic monitoring of nephrotoxic antibiotics in surgical intensive care patients. J Trauma 1989; 29:1462–1468; discussion 8–70.

11. Rybak MJ, Abate BJ, Kang SL, et al. Prospective evaluation of the effect of an aminoglycoside dosing regimen on rates of observed nephrotoxicity and ototoxicity. Antimicrob Agents Chemother 1999; 43:1549–1555.

12. Moise PA, Forrest A, Bhavnani SM, et al. Area under the inhibitory curve and a pneumonia scoring system for predicting outcomes of vancomycin therapy for respiratory infections by *Staphylococcus aureus*. Am J Health Syst Pharm 2000; 57(suppl 2):S4–S9.

13. Fagon J, Patrick H, Haas DW, et al. Treatment of gram-positive nosocomial pneumonia. Prospective randomized comparison of quinupristin/dalfopristin versus vancomycin. Nosocomial Pneumonia Group. Am J Respir Crit Care Med 2000; 161:753–762.

14. Malangoni MA, Crafton R, Mocek FC. Pneumonia in the surgical intensive care unit: factors determining successful outcome. Am J Surg 1994; 167:250–255.

15. Khatib R, Riederer KM, Held M, et al. Protracted and recurrent methicillin-resistant *Staphylococcus aureus* bacteremia despite defervescence with vancomycin therapy. Scand J Infect Dis 1995; 27:529–532.

16. Gonzalez C, Rubio M, Romero-Vivas J, et al. Bacteremic pneumonia due to *Staphylococcus aureus*: a comparison of disease caused by methicillin-resistant and methicillin-susceptible organisms. Clin Infect Dis 1999; 29:1171–1177.

17. Hyatt JM, McKinnon PS, Zimmer GS, et al. The importance of pharmaco-kinetic/pharmacodynamic surrogate markers to outcome. Focus on antibacterial agents. Clin Pharmacokinet 1995; 28:143–160.

18. Sakoulas G, Moise-Broder PA, Schentag J, et al. Relationship of MIC and bactericidal activity to efficacy of vancomycin for treatment of methicillin-resistant *Staphylococcus aureus* bacteremia. J Clin Microbiol 2004; 42:2398–2402.

19. Lodise TP, Graves J, Evans A, et al. Relationship between vancomycin MIC and failure among patients with methicillin-resistant *Staphylococcus aureus* bacteremia treated with vancomycin. Antimicrob Agents Chemother 2008; 52:3315–3320.

20. Performance Standards for Antimicrobial Susceptibility Testing. Sixteenth informational supplement. Wayne, PA: Clinical and Laboratory Standards Institute/NCCLS; 2006. Report No.: M100-S16.

21. FDA alert: FDA lowers vancomycin breakpoints for *Staphylococcus aureus*. Infectious Diseases Society of America, 2009. Available at: http://www.idsociety.org/Content.aspx?id=11378. Accessed June 27, 2009.

22. Vancomycin injection, USP in GALAXY plastic container (PL 2040) for intravenous use only (package insert). Baxter Healthcare Corporation, 2009. Available at: http://www.accessdata.fda.gov/drugsatfda_docs/label/2009/050671s014lbl.pdf. Accessed June 27, 2009.

23. Cruciani M, Gatti G, Lazzarini L, et al. Penetration of vancomycin into human lung tissue. J Antimicrob Chemother 1996; 38:865–869.

24. Daschner FD, Frank U, Kummel A, et al. Pharmacokinetics of vancomycin in serum and tissue of patients undergoing open-heart surgery. J Antimicrob Chemother 1987; 19:359–362.

25. Guidelines for the management of adults with hospital-acquired, ventilator-associated, and healthcare-associated pneumonia. Am J Respir Crit Care Med 2005; 171:388–416.

26. Hidayat LK, Hsu DI, Quist R, et al. High-dose vancomycin therapy for methicillin-resistant *Staphylococcus aureus* infections: efficacy and toxicity. Arch Intern Med 2006; 166:2138–2144.

27. Jeffres MN, Isakow W, Doherty JA, et al. Predictors of mortality for methicillin-resistant *Staphylococcus aureus* health-care-associated pneumonia: specific evaluation of vancomycin pharmacokinetic indices. Chest 2006; 130:947–955.

28. Woodford N. Biological counterstrike: antibiotic resistance mechanisms of Gram-positive cocci. Clin Microbiol Infect 2005; 11(suppl 3):2–21.

29. Sievert DM, Rudrik JT, Patel JB, et al. Vancomycin-resistant *Staphylococcus aureus* in the United States, 2002–2006. Clin Infect Dis 2008; 46:668–674.

30. Levine DP, Fromm BS, Reddy BR. Slow response to vancomycin or vancomycin plus rifampin in methicillin-resistant *Staphylococcus aureus* endocarditis. Ann Intern Med 1991; 115:674–680.

31. Wysocki M, Delatour F, Faurisson F, et al. Continuous versus intermittent infusion of vancomycin in severe staphylococcal infections: prospective multicenter randomized study. Antimicrob Agents Chemother 2001; 45:2460–2467.

32. Conte JE Jr., Golden JA, Kipps J, et al. Intrapulmonary pharmacokinetics of linezolid. Antimicrob Agents Chemother 2002; 46:1475–1480.

33. Honeybourne D, Tobin C, Jevons G, et al. Intrapulmonary penetration of linezolid. J Antimicrob Chemother 2003; 51:1431–1434.

34. Honeybourne D, Tobin C, Jevons G, et al. Erratum: intrapulmonary penetration of linezolid. J Antimicrob Chemother 2003; 52:536.

35. Gee T, Ellis R, Marshall G, et al. Pharmacokinetics and tissue penetration of linezolid following multiple oral doses. Antimicrob Agents Chemother 2001; 45:1843–1846.

36. ZYVOX® (linezolid) injection, (linezolid) tablets, (linezolid) for oral suspension. Pharmacia & Upjohn Company, Division of Pfizer Inc., 2009. Available at: http://media.pfizer.com/files/products/uspi_zyvox.pdf. Accessed June 28, 2009.

37. Mendelson MH, Hartman CS, Wang Y, et al. Evaluation of potential drug interactions of linezolid with selective serotonin reuptake inhibitors (SSRIs) and other antidepressants: analysis of phase 3 and 4 clinical trials [poster presentation]. Washington, DC., 2005.

38. Soriano A, Miro O, Mensa J. Mitochondrial toxicity associated with linezolid. N Engl J Med 2005; 353:2305–2306.

39. Peppard WJ, Weigelt JA. Role of linezolid in the treatment of complicated skin and soft tissue infections. Expert Rev Anti Infect Ther 2006; 4:357–366.

40. Mendes RE, Deshpande LM, Castanheira M, et al. First report of *cfr*-mediated resistance to linezolid in human staphylococcal clinical isolates recovered in the United States. Antimicrob Agents Chemother 2008; 52:2244–2246.

41. Meka VG, Gold HS. Antimicrobial resistance to linezolid. Clin Infect Dis 2004; 39:1010–1015.

42. Paterson DL, Harrison LH, Linden PK, et al. Susceptibility of vancomycin resistant *Entercoccus faecium* (VRE) to quinopristin/dalfopristin (Q/D), linezolid (LZD), and daptomycin [abstract K-1409]. 43rd Interscience Conference on Antimicrobial Agents and Chemotherapy. Chicago: American Society for Microbiology, 2003:386.

43. Weigelt JA. A comparison of ampicillin/sulbactam and cefoxitin in the treatment of bacterial skin and skin-structure infections. Adv Ther 1994; 11:183–191.

44. Itani KM, Weigelt J, Li JZ, et al. Linezolid reduces length of stay and duration of intravenous treatment compared with vancomycin for complicated skin and soft tissue infections due to suspected or proven methicillin-resistant *Staphylococcus aureus* (MRSA). Int J Antimicrob Agents 2005; 26:442–448.

45. Cubicin package insert. Cubist Pharmaceuticals, Inc., 2009. Available at: http://www.cubicin.com/pdf/PrescribingInformation.pdf. Accessed June 28, 2009.

46. Fowler VG Jr., Boucher HW, Corey GR, et al. Daptomycin versus standard therapy for bacteremia and endocarditis caused by *Staphylococcus aureus*. N Engl J Med 2006; 355:653–665.

47. Cubist Pharmaceuticals announces results from first pPhase III Cidecin® community-acquired pneumonia trial comtex, 2002. Available at: http://www.corporate-ir.net/ireye/ir_site.zhtml?ticker=CBST&script=460&layout=6&item_id=247302. Accessed August 15, 2006.

48. Silverman JA, Mortin LI, Vanpraagh AD, et al. Inhibition of daptomycin by pulmonary surfactant: in vitro modeling and clinical impact. J Infect Dis 2005; 191:2149–2152.

49. Munoz-Price LS, Lolans K, Quinn JP. Emergence of resistance to daptomycin during treatment of vancomycin-resistant *Enterococcus faecalis* infection. Clin Infect Dis 2005; 41:565–566.

50. Lewis JS, 2nd, Owens A, Cadena J, et al. Emergence of daptomycin resistance in *Enterococcus faecium* during daptomycin therapy. Antimicrob Agents Chemother 2005; 49:1664–1665.

51. Skiest DJ. Treatment failure resulting from resistance of *Staphylococcus aureus* to daptomycin. J Clin Microbiol 2006; 44:655–656.

52. Cui L, Tominaga E, Neoh HM, et al. Correlation between reduced daptomycin susceptibility and vancomycin resistance in vancomycin-intermediate *Staphylococcus aureus*. Antimicrob Agents Chemother 2006; 50:1079–1082.

53. Silverman JA, Oliver N, Andrew T, et al. Resistance studies with daptomycin. Antimicrob Agents Chemother 2001; 45:1799–1802.

54. Tigacil package insert. Wyeth Pharmaceuticals, Inc., 2009. Available at: http://www.wyeth.com/content/showlabeling.asp?id=491. Accessed June 28, 2009.

55. Kaka AS, Rueda AM, Shelburne SA III, et al. Bactericidal activity of orally available agents against methicillin-resistant *Staphylococcus aureus*. J Antimicrob Chemother 2006; 58:680–683.

56. Markowitz N, Quinn EL, Saravolatz LD. Trimethoprim-sulfamethoxazole compared with vancomycin for the treatment of *Staphylococcus aureus* infection. Ann Intern Med 1992; 117:390–398.

57. Ruhe JJ, Monson T, Bradsher RW, et al. Use of long-acting tetracyclines for methicillin-resistant *Staphylococcus aureus* infections: case series and review of the literature. Clin Infect Dis 2005; 40:1429–1434.

58. Lewis JS II, Jorgensen JH. Inducible clindamycin resistance in staphylococci: should clinicians and microbiologists be concerned? Clin Infect Dis 2005; 40:280–285.

59. Lin SW, Carver PL, DePestel DD. Dalbavancin: a new option for the treatment of gram-positive infections. Ann Pharmacother 2006; 40:449–460.

60. Jauregui LE, Babazadeh S, Seltzer E, et al. Randomized, double-blind comparison of once-weekly dalbavancin versus twice-daily linezolid therapy for the treatment of complicated skin and skin structure infections. Clin Infect Dis 2005; 41:1407–1415.

61. Stryjewski ME, O'Riordan WD, Lau WK, et al. Telavancin versus standard therapy for treatment of complicated skin and soft-tissue infections due to gram-positive bacteria. Clin Infect Dis 2005; 40:1601–1607.

62. Stryjewski ME, Chu VH, O'Riordan WD, et al. Telavancin versus standard therapy for treatment of complicated skin and skin structure infections caused by gram-positive bacteria: FAST 2 study. Antimicrob Agents Chemother 2006; 50:862–867.

63. McKay GA, Beaulieu S, Arhin FF, et al. Time-kill kinetics of oritavancin and comparator agents against *Staphylococcus aureus*, *Enterococcus faecalis* and *Enterococcus faecium*. J Antimicrob Chemother 2009; 63:1191–1199.

64. Anderson DL. Oritavancin for skin infections. Drugs Today (Barc) 2008; 44:563–575.

65. Crandon J, Nicolau DP. Oritavancin: a potential weapon in the battle against serious gram-positive pathogens. Future Microbiol 2008; 3:251–263.

66. Jones ME. In-vitro profile of a new beta-lactam, ceftobiprole, with activity against methicillin-resistant *Staphylococcus aureus*. Clin Microbiol Infect 2007; 13(suppl 2):17–24.

67. Jones RN, Deshpande LM, Mutnick AH, et al. In vitro evaluation of BAL9141, a novel parenteral cephalosporin active against oxacillin-resistant staphylococci. J Antimicrob Chemother 2002; 50:915–932.

68. Chambers HF. Ceftobiprole: in-vivo profile of a bactericidal cephalosporin. Clin Microbiol Infect 2006; 12(suppl 2):17–22.

69. Chambers HF. Evaluation of ceftobiprole in a rabbit model of aortic valve endocarditis due to methicillin-resistant and vancomycin-intermediate *Staphylococcus aureus*. Antimicrob Agents Chemother 2005; 49:884–888.

70. Appelbaum PC, Jacobs MR. Recently approved and investigational antibiotics for treatment of severe infections caused by Gram-positive bacteria. Curr Opin Microbiol 2005; 8:510–517.

71. Appelbaum PC. MRSA—the tip of the iceberg. Clin Microbiol Infect 2006; 12(suppl 2):3–10.

72. Bogdanovich T, Clark C, Ednie L, et al. Activities of ceftobiprole, a novel broad-spectrum cephalosporin, against Haemophilus influenzae and Moraxella catarrhalis. Antimicrob Agents Chemother 2006; 50:2050–2057.

73. Bogdanovich T, Ednie LM, Shapiro S, et al. Antistaphylococcal activity of ceftobiprole, a new broad-spectrum cephalosporin. Antimicrob Agents Chemother 2005; 49:4210–4219.

74. Goldstein EJ, Citron DM, Merriam CV, et al. In vitro activity of ceftobiprole against aerobic and anaerobic strains isolated from diabetic foot infections. Antimicrob Agents Chemother 2006; 50:3959–3962.

75. Livermore DM. Can beta-lactams be re-engineered to beat MRSA? Clin Microbiol Infect 2006; 12(suppl 2):11–16.

76. Noel GJ, Bush K, Bagchi P, et al. A randomized, double-blind trial comparing ceftobiprole medocaril with vancomycin plus ceftazidime for the treatment of patients with complicated skin and skin-structure infections. Clin Infect Dis 2008; 46:647–155.

77. Nicholson SC, Strauss RA, Michiels B, et al. Efficacy of ceftobiprole (BPR) compared to ceftriaxone (CTX) +/− linezolid (L) for the treatment of hospitalized community-acquired pneumonia (poster board #C16). American Thoracic Society International Conference, Toronto, Ontario, Canada, 2008: A677.

78. Talbot GH, Thye D, Das A, et al. Phase 2 study of ceftaroline versus standard therapy in treatment of complicated skin and skin structure infections. Antimicrob Agents Chemother 2007; 51:3612–3616.

79. Hawser S, Lociuro S, Islam K. Dihydrofolate reductase inhibitors as antibacterial agents. Biochem Pharmacol 2006; 71:941–948.

80. Peppard WJ, Schuenke CD. Iclaprim, a diaminopyrimidine dihydrofolate reductase inhibitor for the potential treatment of antibiotic-resistant staphylococcal infections. Curr Opin Investig Drugs 2008; 9:210–225.

81. Jones RN, Biedenbach DJ, Sader HS. In vitro activity of iclaprim and comparison agents tested against Neisseria gonorrhoeae including medium growth supplement effects. Diagn Microbiol Infect Dis 2009; 63:339–341.

82. Arpida publishes top-line data of phase II "intravenous-to-oral" switch trial with oral iclaprim. Arpida Ltd Headquarters, Research and Development, 2008. Available at: http://www.arpida.ch/index.php?NewsID=35&UserID=1. Accessed June 30, 2009.

83. Efficacy/safety of iclaprim in patients with complicated skin infections shown by phase III data, 2008. Available at: www.medicalnewstoday.com/articles/127030.php. Accessed June 30, 2009.

Gram-Positive Resistance—
Clinical Implications

John C. Rotschafer, Mary A. Ullman, and Isaac Mitropoulos
Department of Experimental and Clinical Pharmacology, College of Pharmacy,
University of Minnesota, Minneapolis, Minnesota, U.S.A.

INTRODUCTION

Throughout the modern antibiotic era, *Staphylococcus aureus* has remained a formidable and adaptable pathogen. Through the production of penicillinase, *S. aureus* has averted the effect of penicillin G and congeners (1). Through a penicillin-binding protein 2 alteration (PBP-2a), the pathogen has overcome semisynthetic penicillins and first-generation cephalosporins (2). Infections caused by this altered form of *S. aureus* have been shown to cause increased morbidity and mortality and are more expensive to care for than methicillin-susceptible *S. aureus* (MSSA) strains (3). While often referred to as methicillin-resistant *S. aureus* (MRSA), this term does not reflect contemporary susceptibility testing procedures that are now performed with oxacillin not methicillin, so the more suitable term would be oxacillin-resistant *S. aureus* (ORSA) (4). Some investigators have promoted cefoxitin as the best β-lactam substrate for identifying *S. aureus* with a PBP-2a and a cefoxitin disk along with an oxacillin minimum inhibitory concentration (MIC) is recommend by the CLSI as the standard testing procedure for MRSA/ORSA (4). Additionally, the presence of MRSA can now be confirmed using various gene probe tests that determine the presence of *mec*A, the gene responsible for the alteration of PBP-2. Borderline-resistant *S. aureus* (BORSA) are hyper-β-lactamase–producing strains that are *mec*A negative and can be misinterpreted to be MRSA in antibiotic susceptibility testing (2).

Vancomycin, which for years has been the gold standard antibiotic for the management of MRSA infections was actually named "vanco" with the expectation that the drug would "vanquish" penicillinase-producing strains of *S. aureus* seen in the late 1940s and early 1950s (5–8). While vancomycin has been a mainstay drug for approximately 50 years, reports of vancomycin or glycopeptide intermediate *S. aureus* (VISA/GISA), vancomycin-resistant *S. aureus* (VRSA), heteroresistant strains (h-VISA), and now the suggestion of an MIC creep suggest signs of the drug's aging and the need for a possible replacement (9–11).

Over time, *S. aureus* has also developed a number of other mechanisms or genetic changes to help thwart the effect of modern antibiotic therapy. Many staphylococci will produce glycocalyx or biofilm. Glycocalyx can create an additional barrier to antibiotic penetration, slowing or limiting the desired antibiotic effect. Glycocalyx may also limit the availability of nutrients, slowing the bacterial metabolic growth rate and putting the pathogen in stationary growth. As most antibiotics function as metabolic poisons, a reduction in the bacterial growth rate compromises or eliminates the antibiotic effect. Glycocalyx also interferes with *Staphylococcus* white blood cell phagocytosis by covering bacterial cell wall surface receptors.

Recent reports have identified the accessory gene regulator (agr) as a controller of staphylococcal virulence (12). Polymorphism of the *agr* gene has been reported to alter pathogenicity of *S. aureus* (12). Slow-growing staphylococcal microcolony variants have been reported with infections such as chronic osteomyelitis that are resilient to antibiotic therapy, again likely because of the reduced metabolic rate, making the organism less susceptible to antibiotics.

Sabath and colleagues years ago reported the phenomena of bacterial tolerance in staphylococci (13). Instead of the expected bactericidal and lytic effect associated with cell wall–active antibiotics such as the penicillins or vancomycin, bacteria continue to survive. Early theories suggested that tolerance was the result of an overproduction of autolysin inhibitor that prevented the staphylococci from initiating autolysis after being damaged by cell wall–active antibiotics.

MRSA especially community-acquired MRSA (CA-MRSA) are capable of significant toxin production, including super antigens (14). Most CA-MRSA produce Panton-Valentine leukocidin (PVL) toxin. This toxin has been promoted as a method to distinguish CA-MRSA from hospital-acquired MRSA (HA-MRSA). CA-MRSA and HA-MRSA also differ in the *mec*A subset of the staphylococcal cassette chromosome (SCC). CA-MRSA tend to be type 4 or 5 while HA-MRSA tend to be type 2 (14). While the presence of PVL and/or SCC*mec*A type 4 are highly suggestive of CA-MRSA, there can be an overlap with HA-MRSA (14). Thus, the presence of these features, while highly suggestive, is not a definitive method to identify CA-MRSA.

Generally by the time a patient presents to their physician with signs and symptoms of infection, there is already a significant bacterial burden present and possibly lethal amounts of staphylococcal toxin already produced. Regardless of the speed or the effect cell wall antibiotics may have in killing staphylococci, the release of stored toxin can still have a devastating effect on the patient's clinical course and survival. Use of antibiotics that target protein synthesis such as clindamycin and do not lyse the bacteria may shut down further bacterial toxin synthesis and limit or prevent the release of stored toxin.

Lastly, CA-MRSA appears to have a different antibiotic susceptibility profile as compared to HA-MRSA in that antibiotics such as clindamycin, trimethoprim/sulfamethoxazole, and minocycline/doxycycline can successfully be used to treat patients infected with this pathogen (15). Unfortunately, the antibiotic susceptibility profile also seems to be changing with time for CA-MRSA. Approximately 30% of CA-MRSA exhibit inducible clindamycin resistance and the fluoroquinolone class susceptibility is rapidly being lost as well (14,16).

Historically, the pharmaceutical industry was introducing a sufficient number of new, innovative antibiotics to outpace the bacteria's ability to develop resistance. Because of several major pharmaceutical companies abandoning antibiotic development and the fact that antimicrobials are not as economically attractive to the industry as developing new maintenance drugs, practicing clinicians all too often find themselves looking for an unavailable antibiotic alternative. To call public attention to this dilemma, the Infectious Disease Society of America (IDSA) began in 2004, promoting a program "Bad Bugs, No Drugs." The IDSA position was updated in 2009 with the release of the "Bad Bugs, No Drugs, No ESKAPE" statement (17). While on the gram-negative side the picture is bleak, for gram positives there are a number of new agents in development although in 2008 the Food and Drug Administration (FDA) approved no new antibiotics.

The purpose of this chapter will be to examine underlying mechanisms of bacterial resistance; that is, how gram-positive bacteria use these strategies to overcome the effect of antibiotic therapy.

MECHANISMS OF ANTIBIOTIC RESISTANCE—β-LACTAMS

Bacteria usually overcome the effect of an antibiotic by preventing intracellular access (porin channel blockade), pumping the antibiotic from inside the cell back into the environment (efflux), enzyme inactivation, alteration of the antibiotic target site, blockade of the antibiotic binding site, or overcoming the blockade of a critical metabolic pathway. Depending on the pathogen, multiple mechanisms of resistance may exist simultaneously. For *S. aureus*, enzyme inactivation and target alteration are the two primary mechanisms associated with resistance to β-lactam antibiotics.

β-Lactamase is a generic term referring to enzymes capable of opening the signature β-lactam ring of this class of antibiotics and rendering the antibiotic biologically inactive. The enzyme is a protein made up of amino acids, and the order of this amino acid sequence determines the enzyme's spectrum and potency. The first and most commonly reported β-lactamase was named TEM-1 with the first three letters coming from the name of the patient where the enzyme-producing bacteria was isolated. The next recognized group of β-lactamases were termed SHV (sulfhydryl variant).

The so-called extended spectrum β-lactamases (ESBLs) are a group of enzymes closely related to TEM-1, TEM-2, and SHV-1 but usually differ by a small number of amino acid substitutions. As a result, the ESBL enzymes have a broader substrate spectrum and are more potent. There are now several hundred reported β-lactamases and several classification schemes that have been used that are beyond the scope of this review.

Depending on the specific enzyme, the substrate preference may be a penicillin or cephalosporin making the enzyme a penicillinase or cephalosporinase although there are enzymes capable of hydrolyzing both substrates. Carbapenemases are broad-spectrum enzymes that essentially wipe out the entire β-lactam class including penem antibiotics (imipenem, meropenem, ertapenem, and doripenem) but have not been reported with *S. aureus*. Generally, the clinical strategy is to use a semisynthetic penicillin or cephalosporin that has been chemically altered to preserve the integrity of the β-lactam ring from enzymatic attack or to use a β-lactam/ β-lactamase inhibitor combination (BLIC), ampicillin/sulbactam, amoxicillin/clavulanate, or piperacillin/tazobactam. The enzyme inhibitors such as sulbactam, clavulanate, or tazobactam are also β-lactam drugs but designed to have a greater affinity for the β-lactamase than the β-lactam to which the drug is paired. The β-lactamase inhibitor functions either as a competitive or suicide inhibitor sacrificing itself as a preferred enzyme substrate to protect the paired β-lactam antibiotic from enzymatic attack.

MECHANISMS OF ANTIBIOTIC RESISTANCE—VANCOMYCIN

True vancomycin resistance (VRSA) although reported has been relatively rare (18–20). The mechanism of resistance relates to the *S. aureus* being able to assimilate a vancomycin-resistant enterococcal plasmid, usually vanA, which makes the pathogen resistant to the effects of vancomycin by altering the two terminal amino acids (D-ala-D-ala) used to create the pentapeptide; *S. aureus* uses this pentapetide to crosslink the cell wall (21). This alteration in the two-terminal amino acid sequence (D-ala-D-lac or D-ala-D-ser with other phenotypes) greatly reduces vancomycin binding, causing resistance. The mechanism of vancomycin or glycopeptide intermediate-resistant *S. aureus* (VISA/GISA) is not clear but seems to relate to the reported thickening of the cell wall that is thought to reduce vancomycin penetration or results in the trapping of the antibiotic in the inner cell wall.

Clinicians should be aware that the Clinical and Laboratory Standards Institute (CLSI formerly NCCLS) changed vancomycin breakpoints for *S. aureus* in 2006 (22,23). Previously, the MIC breakpoint for vancomycin-sensitive strains was ≤4 mg/L, for intermediate (VISA/GISA) was 8 to 16 mg/L, and for resistance (VRSA) was ≥32 mg/L. The redefined vancomycin breakpoints reduce each parameter by one doubling dilution, so sensitive is now ≤2 mg/L, intermediate is 4 to 8 mg/L, and resistant is ≥16 mg/L. As a result of this CLSI action, VRSA and VISA/ GISA have been redefined comparing the periods of pre-2006 versus post-2006.

An ominous development for vancomycin is the reporting of vancomycin-heteroresistant strains of *S. aureus* (h-VISA), which appears to be much more common than VRSA or GISA/VISA (24–26). While the mechanism of this form of resistance is not well defined, using vancomycin to manage infections caused by h-VISA strains seems to adversely alter the expected clinical and microbiologic outcome. Heteroresistance is somewhat of a misnomer, as by CLSI definition a vancomycin MIC of ≤2 mg/L for *S. aureus* is by definition a sensitive pathogen. Clinically, however, *S. aureus* with vancomycin MIC values of 1, 1.5, or 2 mg/L are considered likely h-VISA strains. There are definitive E-test methods or population analysis methods to identify h-VISA, but clinical laboratories will likely not be performing these tests;

so vancomycin MICs of 1, 1.5, or 2 mg/L will serve as surrogate markers for h-VISA (27). Vancomycin MIC values may differ depending on the method used to generate the value. Differences in vancomycin MIC have been reported between different automated systems and manual methods (28). Vancomycin MIC can also be affected by the inoculum size used in the test or whether testing is done aerobically or anaerobically (29,30). While testing with a larger inocula or using anaerobic conditions does not reflect standard CLSI methods, they may be more representative of the local environment at the site of infection with this facultative pathogen.

The nature of reporting vancomycin MIC values with automated systems may have stealthed clinician awareness of h-VISA. Automated systems used for reporting vancomycin MIC values such as Vitek and Microscan reported all values under 1 mg/L as ≤1 mg/L for Vitek and all MIC values under 2 mg/L as ≤2 mg/L for Microscan, making detection of *S. aureus* with these higher but that of "sensitive" vancomycin MICs impossible. Both reporting systems have now recalibrated their reporting so that this is no longer an issue, providing the laboratory has the correct software and testing cards.

MECHANISMS OF ANTIBIOTIC RESISTANCE—CLINDAMYCIN

While clindamycin is not used in the management of HA-MRSA, the drug has been used to manage CA-MRSA and inducible MLS$_b$ resistance has been reported, which requires clinicians wishing to use clindamycin to have the laboratory perform a D-test to determine if inducible resistance is present. This test requires that the technician place both an erythromycin and clindamycin disk on an agar plate inoculated with the *S. aureus* in question. If induction is in play, erythromycin will induce the expression of this phenomenon as the antibiotics migrate between the two disks. In a susceptible situation, the clindamycin will result in a symmetric circular zone of inhibition surrounding the disk. In situations where induction is present, the area between the two antibiotic disks becomes blunted, producing a "D" shape instead of an "O" shape surrounding the clindamycin disk, hence the name. Patel et al. have reported that the overall prevalence of inducible clindamycin resistance was 52% in 402 isolates of *S. aureus* (16).

MECHANISM OF RESISTANCE—LINEZOLID AND DAPTOMYCIN

Jones et al. reported that the MIC-50 and MIC-90 in 1930 MRSA isolates for linezolid were 1 and 2 mg/L and for daptomycin 0.25 and 0.5 mg/L, respectively (31). While antibiotic resistance has been reported for both linezolid and daptomycin, most of the reports involve *Enterococcus*. The apparent underlying mechanism for both staphylococci and enterococci is a reduction in affinity for linezolid at the 50S ribosome through a target site modification in peptidyl transferase in the 23S rRNA.

Recently, however, there was a report identifying an outbreak of linezolid-resistant *S. aureus* (linezolid MIC >8 mg/L) involving 11 patients in a Madrid intensive care unit (32). Average hospital stay for these patients was 34 days and all patients were intubated. There was no description as to the likely mechanism of linezolid resistance.

Early on, many institutions reported staphylococcal isolates with an elevated daptomycin MIC; however, many of these clinical laboratories failed to have the proper concentration of calcium in their testing media, and when the test was repeated at a reference laboratory, the MIC was in the susceptible range. Patel et al. and Boucher et al. have reported that *S. aureus* with elevated vancomycin MIC values may affect daptomycin susceptibility (33,34). Cui et al. report a strong correlation with reduced daptomycin susceptibility and vancomycin resistance in VISA/GISA strains (35). They speculate that the thickened staphylococcal cell wall may impact reduced susceptibility to both drugs. While not a true mechanism of resistance, daptomycin does bind to lung surfactant, and for this reason daptomycin should not be used in the treatment of pneumonia.

EVOLUTION OF VANCOMYCIN IN TIMES OF STAPHYLOCOCCAL RESISTANCE

Over the years, the gold standard for clinical management of hospital MRSA infections has unquestionably been vancomycin. As already noted, MRSA susceptibility to vancomycin may be changing, and there is increasing evidence that infections caused by h-VISA strains may not respond well to vancomycin. Overall, vancomycin is considered a bactericidal (MBC/MIC ratio ≤4) antibiotic, but the rate at which vancomycin kills *S. aureus* and sterilizes the infected site is not impressive.

Levine et al. reported in 42 patients mainly with right-sided endocarditis that on average vancomycin ± rifampin required seven to nine days to sterilize the blood (36). In a more contemporary report, Moise et al. stratified MRSA strains causing bacteremia by vancomycin MIC and reported that the mean time to MRSA eradication was six days when the vancomycin MIC value was 0.5 mg/L, 9.5 days when the vancomycin MIC value was 1 mg/L, and >15 days when the vancomycin MIC was 2 mg/L (37). While vancomycin may be considered a bactericidal (MBC/MIC ratio ≤4) drug by most, Jones et al. reported that 15% of wild-type MRSA were tolerant (MBC/MIC ratio ≥16–32) to the effect of the drug (28).

Sakoulas et al. reported a favorable outcome in 56% of patients with MRSA bacteremia when the vancomycin MIC was 0.5 mg/L but <10% of patients had a favorable outcome when the vancomycin MIC was 1 or 2 mg/L (38). There is also a suggestion in the literature that patients recently exposed to vancomycin may demonstrate reduced susceptibility and increased tolerance to vancomycin with subsequent infections (39). Lodise et al. recently reported their vancomycin susceptibility experience in 92 patients where patients in their experience were most likely to present with a vancomycin MIC of 1, 1.5, or 2 mg/L (40). In stratifying the outcome data for these patients on the basis of whether the MRSA vancomycin MIC was <1.5 or ≥1.5 mg/L, they determined that overall failure and hospital length of stay were significantly higher in the 66 patients with the higher vancomycin MIC values.

Soriano et al. reported that the risk of mortality bordered on being significantly different ($p = 0.08$, OR 2.86) in patients with MRSA bacteremia when the vancomycin MIC was 1.5 mg/L (vs. 1 mg/L) and significantly ($p < 0.001$, OR 6.39) higher when the vancomycin MIC was 2 mg/L (41). These data would suggest that a clinician attempting to manage serious MRSA infections with vancomycin must know the vancomycin MIC value to make an informed decision in using the drug. Serious consideration of alternative agents should be entertained if the pathogen vancomycin MIC is 1.5 or 2 mg/L.

Another development in the use of vancomycin to manage serious MRSA infections has been the various guidelines offered by different organizations regarding treatment of nosocomial or ventilator associated pneumonia, endocarditis, and meningitis. Of note is the departure from the previously recognized range of vancomycin trough concentrations (5–10 mg/L) (42–44). Guidelines now routinely recommend vancomycin troughs of 10 to 15 mg/L or 15 to 20 mg/L. Some limited data suggest that maintaining vancomycin trough concentrations >10 mg/L will help prevent the expression of h-VISA (24,45). Whether these higher vancomycin trough concentrations would be beneficial in infections caused by coagulase-negative staphylococci or enterococci has not been established.

These recommended changes in trough concentrations translate into a need to increase the daily dose of vancomycin by two- to fourfold. Interestingly, despite these guidelines being evidence based, there are no data indicating that these higher vancomycin troughs are more effective or safe. The evidence-based grading of these recommendations is a result of expert opinion not clinical data. As vancomycin has been reported to be a concentration-independent killer of *S. aureus*, there would be no expectation that higher concentrations of vancomycin would produce faster bacterial kill.

Recently published data by Jeffres et al. and Hidayat et al. do not demonstrate better clinical outcomes in patients treated with higher trough concentrations of vancomycin (46,47). A variety of investigators have also reported that with daily doses >4 g, long exposures, or vancomycin trough concentrations (>15 mg/L), there is an increased incidence of patient nephrotoxicity (46–48).

In January of 2009, an interprofessional organization consensus report on the dosing and monitoring of vancomycin was published recommending significantly higher vancomycin doses to produce vancomycin trough concentrations of 15 to 20 mg/L and/or a vancomycin area-under-the-serum-concentration-time curve (AUC/MIC) ratio >400 (49). This document suggested vancomycin loading doses of 25 to 30 mg/kg and maintenance doses of 15 to 20 mg/kg of actual body weight be administered two or three times a day in adult patients with normal renal function. Different Monte Carlo target attainment studies suggest that to achieve an AUC/MIC ratio ≥400, the infecting MRSA must have an MIC of <1 mg/L and daily doses of vancomycin must be at least 3 g to achieve a 90% chance of target attainment (50,51). Many clinicians are uncomfortable using doses of vancomycin of this magnitude, and lower doses may not produce the recommended vancomycin trough concentrations of 15 to 20 mg/L. Also with vancomycin doses ≥15 mg/kg careful consideration should be given as to the use of infusions greater than one hour in duration to prevent red man or red neck syndrome (52,53). Considering previous reports suggesting an increased risk of nephrotoxicity with vancomycin trough concentrations >15 mg/L, patients should be closely monitored to prevent an adverse event.

CONCLUSION

Clearly staphylococci have been in a dynamic state of flux for many years such that the term "*S. aureus*" does not in itself convey enough information as to the diversity of this pathogen and the likely clinical implications. Resistance or heteroresistance to several classes of antibiotics combined with adjunct factors that alter the organism's virulence or further compromises antibiotic therapy is now commonplace with this pathogen. The future ongoing use of vancomycin as the gold standard therapy for MRSA is dubious and at the very least a clinician attempting to use vancomycin to manage an MRSA infection must know the vancomycin MIC of the pathogen.

Unfortunately for the clinician attempting to prospectively manage a *S. aureus* infection, the clinical laboratory is not able to provide critical real time data to make informed management choices. Hospital laboratories will not differentiate HA-MRSA from CA-MRSA, identify bacterial tolerance, indicate the production of glycocalyx, probe agr status, confirm the presence or absence of microcolony variants, and report the vancomycin MIC in a timely manner or report vancomycin steady-state trough concentrations, a priori. *S. aureus* undoubtedly will continue to acclimate to challenging and evolving environments inside and outside of the hospital. These pathogens will continue to confront our ability to successfully intervene and evoke clinical and microbiologic cures. As such our therapy must be equally adaptive and robust to confront this formidable adversary.

REFERENCES

1. Dyke K, Gregory P. Resistance to beta-lactam antibiotics. In: Crossley KB, Archer GL, eds. The Staphylococci in Human Disease. New York: Churchill Livingstone, 1997:139–157.
2. Berger-Bachi B. Resistance not mediated by beta-lactamase (methicillin resistance). In: Crossley KB, Archer GL, eds. The Staphylococci in Human Disease. New York: Churchill Livingstone, 1997:158–174.
3. Lodise T, McKinnon P. Burden of methicillin-resistant *Staphylococcus aureus*: focus on clinical and economic outcomes. Pharmacotherapy 2007; 27:1001–1012.

4. Anon. Performance standards for antimicrobial susceptibility testing, Clinical and Laboratory Standards Institute (CLSI). 2005; M100–S15.
5. Alexander M. A review of vancomycin after 15 years of use. Drug Intell Clin Pharm 1974; 8:520–525.
6. Cooper GL, Given DB. Vancomycin: A Comprehensive Review of 30 Years of Clinical Experience. New York: Park Row Publishers, 1986:84.
7. Geraci J. Vancomycin. Mayo Clin Proc 1977; 52:631–634.
8. Rotschafer JC. Vancomycin. In: Taylor WJ, Diers Caviness MH, eds. A Textbook for the Clinical Application of Therapeutic Drug Monitoring. Irving: Abbott Laboratories, 1986:353–363.
9. Rybak M. Resistance to antimicrobial agents: an update. Pharmacotherapy 2004; 24:203S–215S.
10. Sakoulas G, Moellering R Jr. Increasing antibiotic resistance among methicillin-resistant *Staphylococcus aureus* strains. Clin Infect Dis 2008; 46:S360–S367.
11. Steinkraus G, White R, Friedrich L. Vancomycin MIC creep in non-vancomycin-intermediate *Staphylococcus aureus* (VISA), vancomycin-susceptible clinical methicillin-resistant *S. aureus* (MRSA) blood isolates from 2001–2005. J Antimicrob Chemother 2007; 60:788–794.
12. Moise-Broder PA, Sakoulas G, Eliopoulos GM, et al. Accessory gene regulator group II polymorphism in methicillin-resistant *Staphylococcus aureus* is predictive of failure of vancomycin therapy. Clin Infect Dis 2004; 38:1700–1705.
13. Sabath L, Wheeler, N, Laverdiere M, et al. A new type of penicillin resistance of *S. aureus*. Lancet 1977; 1:443–447.
14. Naimi T, LeDell K, Como-Sabetti K. Comparison of community- and health care-associated methicillin-resistant *Staphylococcus aureus* infection. J Am Med Assoc 2003; 290:2976–2984.
15. Moellering R. Current treatment options for community-acquired methicillin-resistant *Staphylococcus aureus* infection. Clin Infect Dis 2008; 46:1032–1037.
16. Patel M, Waites KB, Moser SA, et al. Prevalence of inducible clindamycin resistance among community and hospital associated *S. aureus* isolates. J Clin Microbiol 2006; 44:2481–2484.
17. Boucher H, Talbot GH, Bradley JS, et al. Bad bugs, no drugs, no ESKAPE! An update from the infectious diseases society of America. Clin Infect Dis 2009; 48:1–12.
18. Anon. Public health dispatch: vancomycin resistant *S. aureus*—Pennsylvania, 2002. MMWR 2002; 51:902.

19. Anon. *S. aureus* resistant to vancomycin—United States, 2002. MMWR 2002; 51:565–566.
20. Anon. Brief report: vancomycin-resistant *S. aureus*—New York. MMWR 2004; 53:322–324.
21. Pootoolal J, Neu J, Wright GD. Glycopeptide antibiotic resistance. Annu Rev Pharmacol Toxicol 2002; 42:381–408.
22. Anon. Performance Standards for Antimicrobial Susceptibility Testing, Clinical and Laboratory Standards Institute (CLSI). 2006; M100–S16.
23. Tenover FC, Moellering RC. The rationale for revising the clinical and laboratory standards institute vancomycin minimal inhibitory concentration interpretive criteria for *S. aureus*. Clin Infect Dis 2007; 44:1208–1215.
24. Howden BP, Johnson PD, Ward PB, et al. Isolates with low-level vancomycin resistance associated with persistent methicillin-resistant *Staphylococcus aureus* bactermia. Antimicrob Agents Chemother 2006; 50:3039–3047.
25. Liu C, Chambers HF. *S. aureus* with heteroresistance to vancomycin: epidemiology, clinical significance, and critical assessment of diagnostic methods. Antimicrob Agents Chemother 2003; 47:3040–3045.
26. Moore M, Perdreau-Remington F, Chambers HF. Vancomycin treatment failure associated with heterogeneous vancomycin intermediate *S. aureus* in a patient with endocarditis and in the rabbit model of endocarditis. Antimicrob Agents Chemother 2003; 47:1262–1266.
27. Wootton M, Howe RA, Walsh T, et al. A modified population analysis profile (PAP) method to detect hetero-resistance to vancomycin in *Staphylococcus aureus* in a UK hospital. J Antimicrob Chemother 2001; 47:399–403.
28. Jones R. Microbiologic features of vancomycin in the 21st century: bactericidal, static activity and applied breakpoints to predict clinical outcomes or detect resistant strains. Clin Infect Dis 2006; 42:S13–S24.
29. LaPlante LK, Rybak MJ. Impact of high-inoculum *Staphylococcus aureus* on the activities of nafcillin, vancomycin, linezolid, and daptomycin, alone and in combination with gentamicin, in an in vitro pharmacodynamic model. Antimicrob Agents Chemother 2004; 48:4665–4672.
30. Larsson A, Walker KJ, Raddatz JK, et al. The concentration independent effect of monoexponential and biexponential decay in vancomycin concentrations on the killing of *S. aureus* under aerobic and anaerobic conditions. J Antimicrob Chemother 1996; 38:589–597.
31. Jones RN, Fritsche T, Sader H, et al. LEADER surveillance program results for 2006: an activity and spectrum analysis of linezolid using clinical isolates

from the United States (50 medical centers). Diagn Microbiol Infect Dis 2007; 59:309–317.

32. De La Torre M, Sanchez, M, Orales. G, et al. Abstract C2-1835a outbreak of linezolid resistant *S. aureus* in intensive care. 46th Annual Meeting of the Interscience Conference on Antimicrobial Agents and Chemotherapy, Washington, D.C., October 28, 2008.

33. Boucher HaS, G. Perspectives on daptomycin resistance, with emphasis on resistance in *S. aureus*. Clin Infect Dis 2007; 45:601–608.

34. Patel J, Levitt LA, Hageman J, et al. An association between reduced susceptibility to daptomycin and reduced susceptibility to vancomycin in *S. aureus*. Clin Infect Dis 2006; 42:1652–1653.

35. Cui L, Tominaga E, Neoh H-M, et al. Correlation between reduced daptomycin susceptibility and vancomycin resistance in vancomycin-intermediate *Staphylococcus aureus*. Antimicrob Agents Chemother 2006; 50:1079–1082.

36. Levine DP, Fromm BS, Reddy BR. Slow response to vancomycin or vancomycin plus rifampin in methicillin-resistant *Staphylococcus aureus* endocarditis. Ann Intern Med 1991; 115:674–680.

37. Moise P, Sakoulas G, Forrest A, et al. Vancomycin in-vitro bactericidal activity and its relationship to efficacy in clearance of methicillin-resistant *S. aureus* bacteremia. Antimicrob Agents Chemother 2007; 51:2582–2586.

38. Sakoulas G, Moise-Broder P, Schentag J, et al. Relationship of MIC and bactericidal activity to efficacy of vancomycin for treatment of methicillin-resistant *S. aureus* bacteremia. J Clin Microbiol 2004; 42:2398–2402.

39. Moise P, Smyth D, El-Fawal N, et al. Microbiological effects of prior vancomycin use in patients with methicillin resistant *S. aureus* bacteremia. J Clin Microbiol 2008; 61:85–90.

40. Lodise T, Graves J, Evans A, et al. Relationship between vancomycin MIC and failure among patients with methicillin-resistant *Staphylococcus aureus* bacteremia treated with vancomycin. Antimicrob Agents Chemother 2008; 52:3315–3320.

41. Soriano A, Marco F, Martinez, et al. Influence of vancomycin minimum inhibitory concentration on the treatment of methicillin resistant *S. aureus* bacteremia. Clin Infect Dis 2008; 46:193–200.

42. America ATSatIDSo. Guidelines for the management of adults with hospital acquired, ventilator-associated, and healthcare-associated Pneumonia. Am J Respir Crit Care Med 2005; 171:388–416.

43. Baddour L, Wilson WR, Bayer AS, et al. Infective endocarditis. Circulation 2005; 111:e394–e433.

44. Tunkel A, Hartman BJ, Kaplan SL, et al. Practice guidelines for the management of bacterial meningitis. Clin Infect Dis 2004; 39:1267–1284.
45. Sakoulas G, Gold HS, Cohen RA, et al. Effects of prolonged vancomycin administration on methicillin-resistant *Staphylococcus aureus* (MRSA) in a patient with recurrent bacteraemia. J Antimicrob Chemother 2006; 57:699–704.
46. Hidayat LK, Hsu DI, Quist R, et al. High-dose vancomycin therapy for methicillin-resistant *Staphylococcus aureus* infections. Arch Intern Med 2006; 166:2138–2144.
47. Jeffres M, Isakow W, Doherty JA, et al. Predictors of mortality for methicillin resistant *S. aureus* healthcare associated pneumonia: specific evaluation of vancomycin pharmacokinetic indices. Chest 2006; 130:947–955.
48. Lodise T, Lomaestro B, Graves J, et al. Larger vancomycin doses (at least four grams per day) are associated with an increased incidence of nephrotoxicity. Antimicrob Agents Chemother 2008; 52:1330–1336.
49. Rybak M, Rotschafer JC, Moellering R Jr., et al. Therapeutic monitoring of vancomycin in adult patients: a consensus review of the American Society of Health-System Pharmacists, the Infectious Diseases Society of America, and the Society of Infectious Diseases Pharmacists. Am J Health-Syst Pharm 2009; 66:82–98.
50. Dowell JA, Goldstein BP, Buckwalter M, et al. Pharmacokinetic-pharmacodynamic modeling of dalbavancin, a novel glycopeptide antibiotic. J Clin Pharmacol 2008; 48:1063–1068.
51. Garcia M, Revilla N, Calvo M, et al. Pharmacokinetic/pharmacodynamic analysis of vancomycin in ICU patients. Intensive Care Med 2007; 33:279–285.
52. Farber B, Moellering RC. Retrospective study of the toxicity of preparations of vancomycin from 1974 to 1981. Antimicrob Agents Chemother 1983; 23:138–141.
53. Newfield PR, Roizen MF. Hazards of rapid administration of vancomycin. Ann Intern Med 1979; 91:581.

Reducing the Risk of Nosocomial Dissemination of Methicillin-Resistant *Staphylococcus aureus*: An Infection Control Perspective

12

Charles E. Edmiston, Jr. and Nathan A. Ledeboer
Department of Surgery and Pathology, Medical College of Wisconsin,
Milwaukee, Wisconsin, U.S.A.

INTRODUCTION

Staphylococcus aureus has been recognized as a major microbial pathogen for well over 100 years, having the capacity to produce a variety of suppurative and toxigenic disease processes (Table 1). Many of these infections are life threatening and have exhibited enhanced virulence in hospitalized patients or individuals with selective risk factors such as diabetes. Within the last 40 years, strains of methicillin-resistant *S. aureus* (MRSA) have rapidly spread throughout the health care environment such that it is estimated 20% to 60% of *S. aureus* isolates recovered from hospitalized patients express methicillin resistance (1). Furthermore, a recent study conducted by the Centers of Disease Control and Prevention (CDC) reported that the rate of hospitalization because of MRSA in the United States was highly variable with the rate for MRSA hospitalization in patients under the age of 14 to be 13.1 per 1000 patient discharges, while the rate for patients above 65 years of age was found to be 63.6 per 1000 patient discharges (2). MRSA has become a significant clinical pathogen in part because of three factors: (*i*) an intrinsic pathogenicity mediated by specific (and often unique) virulence factors, (*ii*) high

TABLE 1   Infections Associated with *Staphylococcus aureus*

Skin and soft tissue wounds
Postoperative surgical site infections
Pneumonia
Osteomylelitis
Septic arthritis
Bacteremia
Endocarditis
Urinary tract
Biomedical device–associated infections

frequency of nosocomial dissemination and acquisition within the health care environment, and (*iii*) limited therapeutic options. Designated strains of hospital-acquired MRSA (HA-MRSA) in addition to expressing resistance to the β-lactam antimicrobial agents are often resistant to other common anti-infectives such as erythromycin, tetracycline, and clindamycin. Recent studies have documented that in addition to increased patient morbidity there is a significant economic burden associated with MRSA infections because of increased length of stay (LOS) and higher related health care costs (3,4).

While the prevalence of MRSA isolates within the hospital environment has increased significantly over the past 30 years, two distinct strains (USA300 and USA400) have emerged as important pathogens in individuals lacking the traditional MRSA risk factors, and are identified as community-associated MRSA (CA-MRSA). The spectrum of disease that are caused by these organisms include skin and soft tissue infections (furuncles, carbuncles, and abscesses) and necrotizing pneumonia (5,6). Unlike hospital-acquired strains of MRSA, CA-MRSA isolates are sensitive to trimethoprim-sulfamethoxazole, gentamicin, tetracycline, and clindamycin; however, selected strains may express an inducible resistance to clindamycin (5,7). While the incidence and clinical significance of CA-MRSA is increasing in the health care environment, it is important from an epidemiologic infection control and treatment perspective to consider these two entities independently, and therefore CA-MRSA are reviewed in a separate chapter of this textbook (chap. 4).

EPIDEMIOLOGY AND PATIENT RISK FACTORS ASSOCIATED WITH MRSA

The gram-positive staphylococci are as a group a major source of patient morbidity in both the hospital and community setting. Table 2 reports the predominant microbial pathogens recovered for hospital-associated bloodstream, surgical site, and respiratory and urinary tract infections on the basis of data obtained from the National Nosocomial Infection Surveillance program administered by the CDC (8–10). Overall, hospital discharges with *S. aureus* infection-related diagnoses are relatively common, and as previously noted, a significant number of hospital-acquired infections associated with *S. aureus* are due to methicillin-resistant strains (20%–60%) (1). In the United States, from 1999 to 2000, the largest percentage of *S. aureus*–related hospitalizations occurred in the southern United States, followed by the midwest, northeast, and west. However, the MRSA-related discharge diagnoses were significantly higher ($p < 0.05$) in the northeast, midwest, and south compared to the western states (2).

A myriad of risk factors have been linked to the acquisition and transmission of MRSA within the hospital environment; these include prolonged hospitalization or admission to a long-term care facility (LTCF), diabetes, peripheral vascular disease, recent antimicrobial therapy, ICU stay, presence of an invasive indwelling device (intravascular or urinary catheter, endotracheal or tracheostomy tube, etc.), and close contact with colonized individuals (11,12). The proportion of MRSA responsible for infection in the critical care patient population has increased from <30% as reported by NNIS in 1989 to 40% in 1997 (9). Furthermore, several reports have indicated that MRSA infections in the

TABLE 2 Predominant Bacterial Pathogens Recovered from Hospital-Associated Infections as Reported from the National Nosocomial Infections Surveillance (NNIS) System Database (8–10)

Source	Microorganism	Percent recovery (%)		
		Hospital wide	MICU	SICU
Bloodstream	CoNS[a]	28	36	36
	S. aureus	16	13	10
	Enterococci	8	16	15
	Candida spp.	8	11	5
	Escherichia coli	6	3	2
	Enterobacter spp.		3	6
Surgical site	*S. aureus*	17		20
	Enterococci	13		8
	CoNS[a]	13		17
	E. coli	9		5
	Ps. seruginosa	8		15
	Enterobacter spp.			1
Respiratory tract	*P. aeruginosa*	17	21	17
	S. aureus	16	20	17
	Enterobacter spp.	10	9	13
	Streptococcus pneumoniae	6		
	H. influenzae	6		
	Klebsiella pneumoniae		8	7
Urinary tract	*E. coli*	25	14	15
	Enterococci	16	14	15
	P. aeruginosa	12	10	13
	Candida spp.	9	31	16
	K. pneumoniae	6		6
	Enterobacter spp.		5	5

[a]CoNS, coagulase-negative staphylococci.

ICU are associated with increased LOS and increased resource utilization (13,14). Specifically, MRSA ventilator-associated pneumonia (VAP) has been documented to independently prolong the duration of ICU hospitalization (15). It is interesting to note that in Scandinavia and the Netherlands the prevalence of HA-MRSA has been less than 1% (13–15). It has been suggested that this low prevalence rate is due in part to a nationwide effort to identify colonized patients combined with strict adherence to institutional isolation policies for managing these colonized individuals.

The role of colonization as a risk factor for subsequent dissemination and infection in the ICU patient has been a controversial subject. One study reported that 13.5% of the admissions to the ICU were associated with a positive culture for MRSA at the time of admission or during ICU hospitalization. The rate of importation of MRSA into the ICU as determined by active surveillance culture was 28.6 per 1000 patient days, while the rate of acquisition once admitted to the ICU was 6.6 per 1000 patient days. Furthermore, 43.8% of these MRSA-positive patients were detected by active surveillance culture (16). Therefore, this study suggests that dissemination of MRSA within the hospital environment is largely an occult process and that importation of MRSA culture–positive (colonized) patients into the ICU is an important step in the horizontal transmission of these organisms among a high-risk patient population. In a separate study, a perspective analysis was performed to investigate risk factors for ICU-acquired MRSA infections in involving ICU and neurologic ICU patients. Nasal cultures were also performed within 48 hours of ICU admission and repeated weekly until colonization was documented or the patient was discharged. A total of 249 patients were followed over a six-month period; 21 MRSA infections (8.4%) were observed during ICU residency (17). Catheter-related bloodstream infections were the most common MRSA-related infection, followed by pneumonia and surgical site infections (SSIs). The authors reported that 59 patients (23%) were positive for MRSA by nasal culture and 12 of these patients (20.3%) developed a subsequent MRSA infection. Using a univariate analysis, duration of ICU residency, intra-abdominal and orthopedic procedures, mechanical ventilation, central venous line insertion, total parenteral nutrition, previous antibiotic usage, nasal MRSA colonization, and the presence of multiple colonized (MRSA) patients in the ICU at the same time were found to be independently associated with MRSA infection.

A recent study from Scotland has suggested that new cases of MRSA in the ICU was strongly associated with staffing (nursing) deficits and failure of basic infection control practices including environmental hygiene. The environmental hygiene component is intriguing since MRSA is rarely viewed as an environmental contaminant like vancomycin-resistant enterococci (VRE) or *Clostridium difficile*. A total of 160 environmental sites (sinks, bedrails, curtains, computer keyboards, etc.) were cultured at selected intervals over a 16-week period. A total of 37 (23%) sites were culture positive for staphylococci, while 26 of the positive cultures (70%) were from sites where frequent hand contact occurred (18). The majority of culture-positive samples revealed coagulase-negative staphylococci; however, in one instance an MRSA isolate recovered from an environmental site was phenotypically similar to a strain recovered independently from two patients. The relationship of understaffing (nursing) practices to the quality of patient care has been clearly addressed in other clinical forums; however, it is interesting to note that a documented nursing deficit coupled with poor housekeeping practices may have served as a catalyst for subsequent MRSA infections within a susceptible (ICU) patient population.

MRSA has become an important cause of postoperative SSIs on all surgical services. However, few reports have identified specific risk factors associated with MRSA infections in surgical patients. One recent study has suggested several postoperative factors that may play a role in the development of an MRSA infection, including discharge to an LTCF, duration of antimicrobial prophylaxis >1 day, and age ≥ 70 years

($p < 0.05$) (19). The LTCF as a risk factor for postoperative infection is likely due to the probable patient exposure to MRSA within an endemic environment such as a nursing home (20). The role of prolonged antibiotic prophylaxis as a postoperative risk factor for MRSA infection is likely more subtle, by suppressing microbial growth within the contaminated wound beyond the period of closure.

A recent study in our laboratory has suggested that microbial contamination of the surgical wound bed in vascular patients is likely a common occurrence and is more problematic during insertion of a biomedical device (21). MRSA device-related infections are associated with high patient morbidity and poor clinical outcomes. In a recent series, MRSA was the single most common pathogen (51.6%) associated with acute-onset vascular graft infections. Mean hospital stay was reported to be longer in MRSA-infected patients compared to a study cohort of vascular patients with postoperative SSIs, and these patients were more likely to undergo an amputation then the cohort group (22). MRSA infection in the vascular patient has been shown to be a significant independent risk factor associated with in-hospital death (23). A recent report from the United Kingdom has suggested that segregation of vascular patients on the basis of active identification of MRSA patients through surveillance cultures or identification of potential risk factors was effective at reducing the rate of MRSA colonization and infection in patients undergoing aortic or lower limb surgery ($p < 0.001$) (24).

In orthopedic patients, MRSA infections in trauma and elective surgical procedures have increased threefold between 1994 and 2001 (25). Preoperative colonization with MRSA has been reported to be a risk factor for subsequent infection. Screening and decolonization of MRSA is therefore viewed as a potential strategy for reducing the risk of postoperative infection in patients undergoing prosthetic implantation (26). The incidence of MRSA infection in liver transplant patients was reported to be 23% with the predominant source of infection to include vascular catheters, surgical wound, abdomen, and lung (27). A mortality rate of

86% was observed for patients with bacteremic pneumonia and other associated risk factors (27). The increased risk of infection and mortality has been linked to the high rate of nasal colonization in patients undergoing orthotopic liver transplantation (27,28). In addition, the presence of large surgical wounds, the use of multiple drains, the routine use of invasive monitoring devices, and impaired granulocytic cell function, all likely enhance the probability of infection with MRSA.

Reports from North America, Europe, and Asia have elevated our concern over the transmission of MRSA between animals and humans. While, MRSA infections in animals have been considered in the past to be rare, strains with genetic similarity to hospital-based isolates are emerging in the equine and domestic pet population (29–32). Using an active surveillance screen strategy, MRSA was recovered from 120 (5.3%) nasal swabs in horses admitted to the Ontario Veterinary College. Clinical infection with MRSA was present or developed in 14 (11.7%) of the horses. Horses that were colonized at the time of admission were more likely to develop clinical MRSA infection than noncolonized horses. The rate of MRSA infection was defined as 1.8 per 1000 admissions (29). The molecular characteristics of selected strains of MRSA recovered from domestic pets have revealed similar phenotypic (antibiogram) and molecular (*mec*A and *erm* genes) characteristics to strains seen in humans (30,31). Studies conducted in Asia have suggested that MRSA strains recovered from both cattle and chickens have some genetic similarity to human strains (32). Finally, a study conducted in a veterinary hospital in the United Kingdom confirms that a potential zoonotic linkage may be occurring between veterinary and human strains of MRSA. Over three hundred swabs were obtained from veterinary staff, hospitalized animals, and environmental surfaces, yielding MRSA from 17.9% of staff members, 9% of the animals, and 10% of the cultured environmental surfaces. Pulse-field gel electrophoresis revealed that 56% of the isolates were genetically similar or identical to one of the two predominant clinical strains found in U.K. hospitals. This study clearly documents the acquisition and dissemination of a clinically significant MRSA strain between humans and pets within a veterinary hospital (33). Transmission of bacterial and viral pathogens from animals to man is not a new concept; however, the role of zoonotic transmission of MRSA is a novel concept for MRSA and one that may likely have potential clinical significance.

LABORATORY DIAGNOSIS AND EARLY DETECTION OF MRSA

MRSA has become a significant clinical pathogen because of its increasing prevalence in the community, significant nosocomial dissemination, frequent treatment failure, and limited therapeutic options (34,35). Consequently, a major financial burden is placed upon the health care system resulting from prolonged hospital stays and more costly therapeutics. Additionally, invasive MRSA infections are responsible for significantly higher morbidity and mortality rates (36–38). Therefore, identifying patients colonized with MRSA and isolating carriers can significantly reduce the incidence of MRSA in a health care setting.

Rapid identification of patients colonized with MRSA may serve to preempt widespread nosocomial dissemination or allow the practitioner to direct appropriate therapy (39). However, universal screening of asymptomatic patients for MRSA colonization remains controversial despite governmental mandates (40,41). Selecting an appropriate patient population for screening, the method for screening, body site screened, and compliance with infection control precautions can influence the potential for reduction in MRSA carriage/infections.

The anterior nares are the most common site of *S. aureus* colonization and the most frequently screened and recommended site because of satisfactory sensitivity and ease in obtaining specimens (38–40). However, recent studies have shown that sampling other body sites (oropharynx, perianal, and groin) may enhance the sensitivity of MRSA screening and predict the likelihood of *S. aureus* infection (42,43). In order to reduce the economic burden related to longer patient stays and higher costs associated with therapy and infection control, rapid and accurate screening tests for MRSA are needed to guide intervention and decrease delays in the implementation of contact precautions. A lengthy specimen turnaround time would further augment the risk of nosocomial transmission; thus, an effective screening protocol is currently deemed to be 24 hours or less.

Traditional methods employed to identify MRSA include standard bacteriological culture such as the utilization of selective and/or differential media. While these methods are the least expensive screening techniques, they result in delayed turnaround time because of the requirement for confirmation of positive results. Traditional methods to screen for MRSA usually employ a selective agar medium (mannitol salt agar with oxacillin or Mueller Hinton agar supplemented with NaCl). Putative positive colonies from these screens are then subcultured to nonselective media (blood agar) for biochemical confirmation and susceptibility testing. Coagulase-positive, gram-positive cocci with a cefoxitin MIC ≥ 8 (or oxacillin MIC ≥ 4) are then identified as MRSA (44). However, identification and susceptibility testing using these methods usually requires multiple subcultures, resulting in a two- to four-day turnaround time, thus significantly reducing the clinical impact of the result.

Newer culture methods used for MRSA detection include the chromogenic media. These media incorporate a chromogen into an agar plate; the chromogen then reacts with an enzyme substrate in *S. aureus*, causing the colony to turn color. The chromogen coupled with an antimicrobial in the media provides a sensitive and specific method to screen for MRSA. Studies evaluating the chromogenic media compared to traditional culture demonstrate excellent sensitivity and specificity with a final result available to the clinician within 24 to 48 hours at a cost marginally higher than traditional culture (45).

Other methods used for MRSA detection, including conventional PCR technology, amplify DNA obtained from clinical isolates by targeting the MRSA-specific *mec*A gene and an *S. aureus* species–specific marker (i.e., *nuc* gene). Conventional PCR requires extensive, meticulous labor that is prone to contamination because of the need for post-PCR processing (46,47). Clearly, traditional bacteriological and conventional PCR methods are time consuming and labor intensive, thus failing to provide information necessary for timely decisions on isolation procedures and effective antimicrobial chemotherapy.

Real-time PCR (RT-PCR) has proven to be an excellent method for the rapid detection of MRSA (48). With rapid turnaround time and exceptional testing accuracy, RT-PCR has proven to be ideal in a clinical setting of moderate MRSA endemicity where large numbers of screens need to be processed on a daily basis (49,50). However, the implementation of RT-PCR in a setting of low endemicity, such as community hospitals, may be unfeasible because of limited work space (i.e., separate rooms for pre-PCR, PCR, and post-PCR work to prevent amplicon contamination), upfront costs, and cost per test (51,52). The expenses and workload of a single PCR exceed the demands of testing one clinical specimen for the presence of MRSA. Therefore, a rapid, accurate, and low-cost screening method that is easily employable in all health care settings would be the next logical step in detecting patients that harbor MRSA.

INFECTION CONTROL INTERVENTIONAL STRATEGIES

MRSA Carriage

The mean prevalence of nasal carriage of *S. aureus* in the United States has been reported to be 32.4%, suggesting that a third of the U.S. population is colonized with *S. aureus*. The community carriage of MRSA was determined to be less than 1.0% (53). However, among individuals who have recently been exposed to selected anti-infectives, the prevalence increases to 4.8%. While asymptomatic colonization with MRSA has been described previously as a risk factor for subsequent MRSA infection, the use of nasal cultures as a screening tool has been viewed as a controversial strategy for reducing the risk (incidence) of MRSA acquisition and dissemination within the hospitalized patient population (40,54). A total of 758 patients admitted to five hospitals were screened for MRSA within 48 hours of admission and during hospitalization using conventional culture methodology. A total of 3.4% of patients harbored MRSA in their nares, 19% of patients colonized with MRSA at admission, and 25% of patients who acquired MRSA during hospitalization developed an infection with MRSA. These results were found to be significant when compared to MSSA-colonized or -noncolonized patients ($p < 0.01$) (54). The study did not assess the impact of colonization as a factor in cross-contamination or nosocomial dissemination of MRSA, but the implications are clear given the wide variance in both adherence to isolation and handwashing policies within U.S. hospitals. The findings suggest that some MRSA-colonized patients while exhibiting no overt symptoms serve as potential reservoirs for dissemination of resistant staphylococci to other high-risk patient populations. A separate prospective, interventional cohort study conducted over a two-year period involving a total of 21,754 surgical patients found that a universal, rapid MRSA admission screening strategy did not reduce the incidence of hospital-acquired MRSA infections within a surgical patient populations (40). In light of the numerous reports in the literature documenting increased risk for infection associated with MRSA-colonized patients admitted to the ICU, several investigator have suggested that screening patients for MRSA colonization prior to ICU admission may be a prudent risk reduction strategy in those high-risk individuals undergoing invasive medical or surgical procedures (12,16,19,20,22,26,27,55,56). Published reports have clearly revealed that an active MRSA surveillance program will uncover previously occult MRSA-colonized patients, leading to an increase in the rate of contact isolation. However, whether or not this type of active (and costly) surveillance program will result in decreased MRSA acquisition and/or overt infection remains unclear (57).

MRSA Patient Isolation

Regardless of the presence or absence of resistant pathogens within the hospital environment, all health care personnel must embrace the fundamental practice of "standard precautions" for all patient populations. Standard precautions imply that all health care professionals will use appropriate hand hygiene, gloves, mask (eye protection), gowns, or other personal protective equipment when they anticipate exposure to blood or body fluid, secretion, excretion, or contact with mucous membranes or nonintact skin. The use of alcohol-based hand rubs have been shown to be effective at reducing hand contamination and increasing hand hygiene compliance, especially within the ICU (58,59) Compliance to hand hygiene policies have been shown to be effective in reducing the rate of nosocomial infections and transmission of MRSA (60,61). Unfortunately, hand hygiene compliance remains poor in many institutions as documented by a recent report in the literature that demonstrated that 85.2% of patient charts in an ICU were contaminated with pathogenic or potentially pathogenic bacterial isolates (62). The contaminating organisms included *Pseudomonas aeruginosa* and *S. aureus*. MRSA was recovered from 6.8% of the outer surface of patient charts in the ICU (63). The authors noted that the high rate of contaminated charts indicated that more emphasis on hand hygiene compliance is required and that inanimate surfaces may also serve as an occult reservoir for resistant nosocomial pathogens.

Patients who are identified as having an MRSA infections are placed in "contact isolation." In addition to "standard precaution," contact isolation prevents the transmission of nosocomially important microbial populations such as MRSA, extended-spectrum β-lactamase-resistant (ESBL) bacteria, selective gram-negative-resistant bacteria, VRE, and *C. difficile*. Patients in "contact isolation" are placed in a private room or cohorted with another patient infected with the same microorganism. Health care worker who enter the patient's room regardless of the reason must wear a gown and gloves prior to entry, removing these article and placing them in an appropriate receptacle upon leaving the room. In addition, appropriate hand hygiene must be practiced after leaving the room and before examining or entering another patient's room. While it has been suggested that isolation policies result in diminished patient care and physician contact, no convincing evidence exists indicating that patients are harmed by our current isolation polices. Alternatively, the evidence suggests that "contact isolation" when coupled with appropriate hand hygiene compliance is effected at reducing the dissemination of resistant pathogens such as MRSA within the health care environment (64,65).

Formulary Considerations

The relationship between antibiotic usage and the rate of MRSA acquisition within the hospital environment has been well documented. The use of broad-spectrum cephalosporins and fluoroquinolones has been associated with both increased rates of colonization and overt infection in susceptible patient populations (66–68). Two case-control studies found a significant relationship between patient exposure to fluoroquinolones and MRSA colonization or infections (67,69). The effective tissue penetration of the fluoroquinolones leads to the eradication of commensal microbial populations, which colonize the skin surfaces, nares, and other mucous membranes, creating a favorable environment for endemic nosocomial populations to repopulate these sites with resistant strains. Attention to antibiotic stewardship is a key consideration in reducing the risk of MRSA within the health care environment. It has been proposed that the emergence of antimicrobial resistant bacterial populations in the intensive care unit can be halted through the process of antibiotic cycling, where the antibiotic formulary is rotated on a 6- to 12-month cycle. Unfortunately, our current understanding of the ecological positioning of microbial populations in the gut or on the surface of the skin suggests a highly complex and intrinsically fluid environment in which antimicrobial cycling by itself will not reduce the burden of antibacterial resistance within the hospital or ICU setting (70). While the perfect strategy is yet to emerge, it is evident that development of a thoughtful and judicious antimicrobial use policy requires a close collegiality between infection control, pharmacy, microbiology, and the clinical staff.

Decolonization

Mupirocin since its introduction 20 years ago has been used successfully by decolonized health care workers who have been implicated in MRSA outbreaks on both the medical and surgical services. Recently, this agent has been used in selective surgical services in combination with active surveillance cultures to identify potential patients colonized with MRSA prior to elective surgical procedures (26,71,72). The use of intranasal mupirocin has also been applied successfully for preventing MRSA infection in the ICU (73). It would appear that mupirocin is effective in eradicating nasal carriage and reducing the risk of infection over the short term; however, the longer-term benefits are presently unknown (74). Furthermore, there are sufficient data to suggest that inappropriate use of mupirocin is associated with emergence (rapid) of resistance, which is highly problematic since mupirocin is currently the only effective agent for MRSA decolonization (75–77).

Reducing the Risk of MRSA Infections within the Hospital Environment

Infections associated with MRSA are problematic since acquisition and dissemination within the hospital environment is often due to failure to adhere to sound, fundamental infection control principles that are relevant to all nosocomial pathogens. In the case of catheter-related bloodstream infection, the cornerstone of preventing CR-BSI is grounded in the basic principles of infection control, judicious handwashing, and aseptic techniques. Rigorous attention to aseptic principles has repeatedly been shown to result in decreased infection. While newer technological developments in the area of wound care and the use of antiseptic/antibiotic impregnated devices have been suggested to reduce the risk of CR-BSI, there is no substitution for meticulous catheter care (78–80). Furthermore, to minimize the risk of contamination, all line insertions must be performed under maximal barrier precautions. This requires using sterile drapes (large), gowns, masks, and gloves. Several prospective studies have demonstrated that a significant reduction in catheter colonization and bacteremia can be achieved using a rigorous aseptic protocol (80). While several surface antiseptics have been used to reduce skin contamination at the insertion site, cleansing with chlorhexidine has been shown to be superior to elemental iodine or an iodophor (80–82). A recent study using a 2% chlorhexidine gluconate (CHG) w/v and 70% isopropyl alcohol (IPA) skin-prepping agent demonstrates superior efficacy when compared with povidone iodine (83). Two points are worth considering: First, chlorhexidine exhibits an excellent residual activity compared to other compounds and second, this agent is not neutralized by blood, serum, or blood proteins (84). Over the past five years there has been a significant national effort to reduce the risk of central line–associated infections through the use of an evidence-based effort, designated as the "central-line bundle," which comprises several key components:

- hand hygiene
- maximal barrier precautions upon insertion
- chlorhexidine skin antisepsis
- optimal catheter site selection, with subclavian vein as the preferred site for nontunneled catheters
- daily review of line necessity with prompt removal of unnecessary lines

S. aureus (MSSA and MRSA) stands out as the most common pathogen associated with pneumonia in the hospital environment. It has been reported that MRSA accounts for up to 14.6% of VAPs (56). In addition, mortality rates related to pneumonia have been reported to be significantly greater among patients with MRSA infection (85,86). One should not underestimate the role that hands play in cross-contamination as a mechanism for transmission of health care–associated pathogens. Cross-contamination has been well documented to occur during tracheal suctioning and manipulation of ventilator circuitry or endotracheal tubes. Therefore, aseptic technique (handwashing) is essential when caring for patients on ventilator support. In addition, it is important to note that devices associated with respiratory therapy or diagnostic examination need to be clean/sterilized/disinfected properly since they may service as a vehicle for dissemination of health care–associated pathogens to at-risk patients. The pathophysiology of VAP follows a rather predictable course beginning with colonization of the airway and tracheal bronchitis; patients often present with acute respiratory distress or sepsis (87,88). Attention to oral hygiene should be viewed as a fundamental component of any effective strategy for reducing the risk of VAP. Finally, head position has been proposed as a simple means for reducing the rate of VAP. A semirecumbent position (30–45°) is associated with a lower risk for VAP compared to patients in a supine position (87).

S. aureus is the most common surgical site pathogen and the incidence of MRSA has increased overall within U.S. hospitals from less than 2.5% in the mid-1970s to greater than 50% in 2003 (89,90). The presence of MRSA in the surgical ICU and other units of the hospital has necessitated the adoption of strict isolation guidelines, which while controversial, have been highly successful in preventing the dissemination and acquisition of these highly virulent organisms within the health care environment (64–66). The management of the surgical wound while intrinsically straightforward is often highly variable from institution to institution. The use of sterile gloves and aseptic technique is well documented for the prevention of wound sepsis during the immediate postoperative period. The CDC has suggested that sterile gloves be used for the first 24 hours of incisional care. However, no specific glove recommendations are offered for the management of postoperative wounds beyond this period. A recent survey found that nurses in acute care facilities were more likely to wear sterile gloves when managing postoperative surgical wounds beyond the 24-hour postoperative window (91). The use of chemically clean versus sterile gloves for managing wounds has emerged as a major discussion point primarily because of the issue of cost. The impact of this strategy on infection control practices within an institution is debatable and subject to individual interpretation. Sterile technique, however, is indicated when managing wounds in immunosuppressed patients or open surgical wounds involving exposed organ/space sites.

There are at present several emerging technologies, which may impact upon infection control practices by reducing the potential for bacterial colonization/contamination of the acute surgical wound. These include the use of dressings that attempt to manipulate the biology of the wound and thereby accelerate normal wound healing. Another strategy has been the incorporation of antimicrobial or antiseptic substances into the matrix of the wound dressing. The incorporation of selected metals such as silver has potential intrinsic value in reducing MRSA contamination within the surgical wounds (92,93). A recent study documented a reduction in MRSA SSIs when a sterile plain gauze dressing was replaced with an antimicrobial dressing impregnated with 0.2% polyhexamethylene biguaide (94). Finally, over the past 15 years numerous antiseptic technologies have been applied to selected biomedical devices (central lines, Foley catheters, shunts, etc.), documenting a reduced risk for selected health care–associated infections in high-risk patient populations. This strategy has been applied to selected braided and monofilament sutures in which these devices are coated with an antiseptic agent (triclosan) (95). The presence of a safe, antiseptic device within the wound bed has great potential benefit, especially in those surgical procedures where the risk of wound contamination is high (96,97). While innovative technology can play an important role in risk reduction, it should only be viewed as an adjunctive component of a comprehensive strategy based on the following surgical cornerstones: timely and appropriate antimicrobial prophylaxis, effective skin antisepsis, and exquisite surgical technique.

Reducing Risk of SSIs on the Front End

A sentinel cornerstone of an effective SSI risk reduction strategy involves the administration of timely and appropriate antimicrobial prophylaxis. Unfortunately, the antistaphylococcal activity of traditional prophylactic agents such as cefazolin (used for clean surgical procedures) has diminished to where approximately 60% of community strains exhibit resistance to this first-generation cephalosporin. While vancomycin remains highly effective against MRSA, prophylactic use of this agent is usually limited to one or more of the following scenarios: a documented allergy to the cephalosporins, MRSA colonization of some body site, the patient has had a previous MRSA infection in lieu of colonization studies, or in a setting where there is a high prevalence of MRSA infections (11,98). Selective strains of CA-MRSA exhibit susceptibility to two older agents, clindamycin and trimethoprim-sulfamethoxazole. These agents may have some clinical utility as prophylactic agents in orthopedic (clindamycin) and urologic surgical procedures (trimethoprim-sulfamethoxazole). Two compounds that have been considered as alternative prophylactic agents in light of their activity against MRSA include linezolide and daptomycin. However, these drugs are viewed as first-line therapeutic agents and routine prophylactic use is strongly discouraged, especially since neither of these agents has been approved by the Centers for Medicare and Medicaid Services for routine antimicrobial prophylaxis.

Finally, an adjunctive strategy that is gaining momentum among surgical practitioners is the use of the preadmission antimicrobial (antiseptic) shower. This strategy involves having the patient take two or more antiseptic showers (skin cleansing) using 2% or 4% CHG prior to hospital admission (99) This simple yet effective procedure deposits a high, persistent concentration of CHG directly to the skin surface, which is significantly higher than the concentration required to inhibit or kill staphylococcal skin flora (drug-sensitive or -resistant strains). The axilla, groin, and perineum are areas of high staphylococcal colonization, which may be a problematic source of contamination during the perioperative period. Therefore, the rationale behind the preadmission shower is to reduce the skin burden of those microbial populations, thereby reducing the risk of SSIs.

FINAL CONSIDERATION—RISK REDUCTION IN A TRANSPARENT ENVIRONMENT

Globally, MRSA infections are a significant cause of patient morbidity and mortality, which is unfortunate since many of these infections could be prevented through careful and thoughtful adherence to basic infection control practices and evidence-based interventional practices. In addition, if we are to reduce the incidence of these infections within the health care setting, all health care professional must be aware of the epidemiology, pathogenesis, and recognized mechanisms of microbial transmission/ acquisition of MRSA and other drug-resistant bacteria. Looming in the not-so-distant future is the specter of compulsory (national) reporting of health care–associated infection rates (100). It will be interesting to note, based on historical trends, what if any impact mandatory reporting of health care–associated infections on a state and national level will have on the overall incidence of MRSA infection in the future (101).

REFERENCES

1. Zinn CS, Westh H, Rosdahl VT. An international multicenter study of antimicrobial resistance and typing of hospital *Staphylococcus aureus* isolates from 21 laboratories in 19 countries or states. Microb Drug Resist 2004; 10:160–168.

2. Kuehnert MJ, Hill HA, Kupronis BA, et al. Methicillin-resistant *Staphylococcus aureus* hospitalizations, United States. Emerg Infect Dis 2005; 11:868–872.

3. Engemann JJ, Carmeli Y, Cosgrove SE, et al. Adverse clinical and economic outcomes attributable to methicillin resistance among patients with *Staphylococcus aureus* surgical site infection. Clin Infect Dis 2003; 36:592–598.

4. Cosgrove SE, Sakoulas G, Perencevich EN, et al. Comparison of mortality associated with methicillin-resistant and methicillin-susceptible *Staphylococcus aureus* bacteremia: a meta analysis. Clin Infect Dis 2003; 36:53–59.

5. Fridkin SK, Hageman JC, Morrison M, et al. Methicillin-resistant *Staphylococcus aureus* disease in three communities. N Engl J Med 2005; 352:1436–1444.

6. Francis JS, Doherty MC, Lopatin U, et al. Severe community-onset pneumonia in healthy adults caused by methicillin-resistant *Staphylococcus aureus* carrying the Panton–Valentine leukocidin genes. Clin Infect Dis 2005; 40:100–107.

7. Lewis JS, Jorgensen JH. Inducible clindamycin resistance in staphylococci: should clinicians and microbiologist be concerned? Clin Infect Dis 2005; 40:280–285.

8. Richards MJ, Edwards JR, Culver DH, et al. Nosocomial infections in medical intensive care units in the United States: National Nosocomial Infections Surveillance System. Crit Care Med 1999; 27:887–892.

9. National Nosocomial Infection Surveillance System. National Nosocomial Infection Surveillance (NIS) System report: data summary from January 1990–May 1999, issued June 1999. Am J Infect Control 1999; 27:520–532.

10. Jarvis WR, Martone W. Predominant pathogens in hospital infections. J Antimicrob Chemother 1992; 29(suppl):19–24.

11. Muto CA, Jernigan JA, Ostrowsky BE, et al. SHEA guideline for preventing nosocomial transmission of multidrug-resistant strains of *Staphylococcus aureus* and *Enterococcus*. Infect Control Hosp Epidemiol 2003; 24:362–386.

12. Marshall C, Wesselingh S, McDonald M, et al. Control of endemic MRSA—what is the evidence? A personal view. J Hosp Infect 2004; 56:253–268.

13. Tiemersma EW, Bronzwaer SL, Lyytikainen O, et al. Methicillin-resistant *Staphylococcus aureus* in Europe, 1999–2002. Emerg Infect Dis 2004; 10:1627–1634.

14. Faria NA, Olivera DC, Westh H, et al. Epidemiology of emerging methicillin-resistant *Staphylococcus aureus* (MRSA) in Denmark: a nationwide

study in a country with low prevalence of MRSA infection. J Clin Microb 2005; 43:1836–1842.

15. Vrien M, Blok H, Fluit A, et al. Cost associated with a strict policy to eradicate methicillin-resistant *Staphylococcus aureus* in Dutch university medical center: a 10 year survey. Eur J Clin Microb Infect Dis 2002; 21: 782–786.

16. Ridenour GA, Wong ES, Call MA, et al. Duration of colonization and methicillin-resistant *Staphylococcus aureus* among patients in the intensive care unit: implications for intervention. Infect Control Hosp Epidemiol 2006; 27:271–278.

17. Oztoprak N, Cevik MA, Korkmaz AF, et al. Risk factors for ICU-acquired methicillin-resistant *Staphylococcus aureus* infections. Am J Infect Control 2006; 34:1–5.

18. Dancer SJ, Coyne M, Speekenbrink A, et al. MRSA acquisition in an intensive care unit. Am J Infect Control 2006; 34:10–17.

19. Manian FA, Meyer L, Setzer J, et al. Surgical site infections associated with methicillin-resistant *Staphyloccus aureus*: do postoperative factors play a role? Clin Infect Dis 2003; 36:863–868.

20. Rezende NA, Blumberg HM, Metzger BS, et al. Risk factors for methicillin-resistance among patients with *Staphylococcus aureus* bacteremia at the time of hospital admission. Am J Med 2002; 323:117–123.

21. Edmiston CE, Seabrook GR, Cambria RA, et al. Molecular epidemiology of microbial contamination in the operating room environment: is there a risk for infections? Surgery 2005; 138:572–588.

22. Taylor MD, Napolitano LM. Methicillin-resistant *Staphylococcus aureus* infections in vascular surgery: increasing prevalence. Surg Infect (Larchmt) 2004; 5:180–188.

23. Cowie SE, Ma I, Lee S, et al. Nosocomial MRSA infection in vascular surgery patients; impact on patient outcome. Vasc Endovascular Surg 2005; 39:327–334.

24. Thompson M. An audit demonstrating a reduction in MRSA infection in a specialized vascular unit resulting from a change in infection control protocol. Eur J Vasc Endovasc Surg 2006; 31:609–615.

25. Nixon M, Jackson B, Varghese P, et al. Methicillin-resistant *Staphylococcus aureus* on orthopaedic wards. J Bone Joint Surg 2006; 88B:812–817.

26. Shams WE, Rapp RP. Methicilin-resistant staphylococcal infections: an important consideration for orthopaedic surgeons. Orthopedics 2004; 27: 565–568.

27. Singh N, Paterson DL, Chang FY, et al. Methicillin-resistant *Staphylococcus aureus*: the other emerging resistant Gram-positive cocci among liver transplant recipients. Clin Infect Dis 2000; 30:322–327.

28. Desai D, Desai N, Nightingale P, et al. Carriage of methicillin-resistant *Staphylococcus aureus* is associated with increased risk of infection after liver transplantation. Liver Transpl 2003; 9:754–759.

29. Weese JS, Rousseau J, Archambault M, et al. Methicillin-resistant *Staphylococcus aueus* in horses at a veterinary teaching hospital: frequency, characterizaton, and associateion with clinical disease. J Vet Intern Med 2006; 20:182–186.

30. Strommenger B, Kehrenbery C, Kettlitz C, et al. Molecular characterization of methicillin-resistant *Staphylococcus aureus* and their relationship to human isolates. J Antimicrob Chemother 2006; 57:461–465.

31. Weese JS, Dick H, Willey BM, et al. Suspected transmission of methicillin-resistant *Staphylococcus aureus* between domestic pets and humans in veterinary clinics and in households. Vet Microbiol 2006; 115:148–155.

32. Lee JH. Occurrence of methicillin-resistant *Staphylococcus aureus* strains from cattle and chickens, and analysis of their *mec*A, *mec*R1 and *mec*I genes. Vet Microbiol 2006; 114:155–159.

33. Loeffler A, Boag AK, Sung J, et al. Prevalence of methicillin-resistant *Staphylococcus aureus* among staff and pets in a small animal referral hospital in the UK. J Antimicrob Chemother 2005; 56:692–697.

34. Leclercq R. Epidemiological and resistance issues in multidrug-resistant staphylococci and enterococci. Clin Microbiol Infect 2009; 15:224–231.

35. Miller LG, Kaplan SL. *Staphylococcus aureus*: a community pathogen. Infect Dis Clin North Am 2009;23:35–52.

36. Naber CK. *Staphylococcus aureus* bacteremia: epidemiology, pathophysiology, and management strategies. Clin Infect Dis 2009; 48:S231–S237.

37. Papia G, Louie M, Tralla A, et al. Screening high-risk patients for methicillin-resistant *Staphylococcus aureus* on admission to the hospital: is it cost effective? Infect Control Hosp Epidemiol 1999; 20:473–477.

38. Struelens MJ, Hawkey PM, French GL, et al. Laboratory tools and strategies for methicillin-resistant *Staphylococcus aureus* screening, surveillance and typing: state of the art and unmet needs. Clin Microbiol Infect 2009; 15: 112–119.

39. Cunningham R, Jenks P, Northwood J, et al. Effect on MRSA transmission of rapid PCR testing of patients admitted to critical care. J Hosp Infect 2007; 65:24–28.

40. Harbarth, S., Fankhauser C, Schrenzel J, et al. Universal screening for methicillin-resistant *Staphylococcus aureus* at hospital admission and nosocomial infection in surgical patients. JAMA 2008; 299:1149–1157.
41. Robicsek A, Beaumont JL, Paule SM, et al. Universal surveillance for methicillin-resistant *Staphylococcus aureus* in 3 affiliated hospitals. Ann Intern Med 2008; 148:409–418.
42. Batra R, Eziefula AC, Wyncoll D, et al. Throat and rectal swabs may have an important role in MRSA screening of critically ill patients. Intensive Care Med 2008; 34:1703–1706.
43. Eveillard, M., de Lassence A, Lancien E, et al. Evaluation of a strategy of screening multiple anatomical sites for methicillin-resistant *Staphylococcus aureus* at admission to a teaching hospital. Infect Control Hosp Epidemiol 2006; 27:181–184.
44. Nahimana I, Francioli P, Blanc DS. Evaluation of three chromogenic media (MRSA-ID, MRSA-Select and CHROMagar MRSA) and ORSAB for surveillance cultures of methicillin-resistant *Staphylococcus aureus*. Clin Microbiol Infect 2006; 12:1168–1174.
45. Carson J, Lui B, Rosmus L, et al. Interpretation of MRSA select screening agar at 24 hours of incubation. J Clin Microbiol 2009; 47:566–568.
46. Information about MRSA for Healthcare Personnel. Centers for Disease Control and Prevention. Available at: www.cdc.gov.
47. Elsayed S, Chow BL, Hamilton NL, et al. Development and validation of a molecular beacon probe-based real-time polymerase chain reaction assay for rapid detection of methicillin resistance in *Staphylococcus aureus*. Arch Pathol Lab Med 2003; 127:845–849.
48. van Hal SJ, Stark D, Lockwood B, et al. Methicillin-resistant *Staphylococcus aureus* (MRSA) detection: comparison of two molecular methods (IDI-MRSA PCR assay and GenoType MRSA Direct PCR assay) with three selective MRSA agars (MRSA ID, MRSASelect, and CHROMagar MRSA) for use with infection-control swabs. J Clin Microbiol 2007; 45:2486–2490.
49. Paule SM, Mehta M, Hacek DM, et al. Chromogenic media vs real-time PCR for nasal surveillance of methicillin-resistant *Staphylococcus aureus*: impact on detection of MRSA-positive persons. Am J Clin Pathol 2009; 131:532–539.
50. Wolk DM, Picton E, Johnson D, et al. Multicenter evaluation of the Cepheid Xpert methicillin-resistant *Staphylococcus aureus* (MRSA) test as a rapid screening method for detection of MRSA in nares. J Clin Microbiol 2009; 47:758–764.

51. Boyce JM, Havill NL. Comparison of BD GeneOhm methicillin-resistant *Staphylococcus aureus* (MRSA) PCR versus the CHROMagar MRSA assay for screening patients for the presence of MRSA strains. J Clin Microbiol 2008; 46:350–351.

52. Buhlmann M, Bögli-Stuber K, Droz S, et al. Rapid screening for carriage of methicillin-resistant *Staphylococcus aureus* by PCR and associated costs. J Clin Microbiol 2008; 46:2151–2154.

53. Mainous AG, Hueston WJ, Everett CJ, et al. Nasal carriage of *Staphylococcus aureus* and methicillin-resistant *S. aureus* in the Unites States, 2001–2002. Ann Fam Med 2006; 4:132–137.

54. Davis KA, Stewart JJ, Crouch HK, et al. Methicillin-resistant *Staphylococcus aureus* (MRSA) nares colonization at hospital admission and its effect on subsequent MRSA infection. Clin Infect Dis 2004; 39:776–782.

55. Cosgrove SE, Qi Y, Kaye KS, et al. The impact of methicillin resistance in *Staphylococcus aureus* bacteremia on patient outcomes: mortality, length of stay and hospital charges. Infect Control Hosp Epidemiol 2005; 26:166–174.

56. Shorr AF, Combes A, Kollef MH. Methicillin-resistant *Staphylococcus aureus* prolongs intensive care unit stay in ventilator-associated pneumonia, despite initially appropriate antibiotic therapy. Crit Care Med 2006; 34:700–706.

57. Warren DK, Guth RM, Coopersmith CM, et al. Impact of a methicillin-resistant *Staphylococcus aureus* active surveillance program on contact precaution untilization in a surgical intensive care unit. Crit Care Med 2007; 35:430–434.

58. Maury E, Alzieu M, Baudel JL, et al. Availability of an alcohol solution can improve hand disinfection compliance in the intensive care unit. Am J Respir Crit Care Med 2000; 162:324–327.

59. Vos A, Widmer AP. No time for handwashing? Handwashing versus alcoholic rub: can we afford 100% compliance? Infect Control Hosp Epidemiol 1997; 18:205–208.

60. Pittel D, Hugonnet S, Harbarth S, et al. Effectiveness of a hospital-wide program to improve compliance with hand hygiene. Lancet 2000; 356:1307–1312.

61. Larson EL. APIC guidelines for handwashing and hand antisepsis in healthcare setting. Am J Infect Control 1995; 23:251–269.

62. Boyce JM, Pittet D. Guidelines for hand hygiene in healthcare setting. Recommendations of the Healthcare Infection Control Practices Advisory Committee and the HICPAC/SHEA/APIC/IDSA Hand Hygiene Task Force. MMWR 2002; 51/RR16:1–56.

63. Pathotra BR, Saxena AK, Al-Mulhim AD. Contamination of patient files in intensive care units: an indication of strict handwashing after entering case notes. Am J Infect Control 2005; 33:398–401.

64. Cooper BS, Stone SP, Kibbler CC, et al. Isolation measures in the hospital management of methicillin-resistant *Staphylococcus aureus* (MRSA): systematic review of the literature. Br Med J 2004; 329:533–541.

65. Boyce JM, Havill NL, Kohan C, et al. Do infection control measures work for methicillin-resistant *Staphylococcus aureus*? Infect Control Hosp Epidemiol 2004; 25:395–401.

66. Henderson DK. Managing methicillin-resistant staphylococci: a paradigm for preventing nosocomial transmission of resistant organisms. Am J Med 2006; 119:S45–S52.

67. Graffunder EM, Venezia RA. Risk factors associated with nosocomial methicillin-resistant *Staphylococcus aureus* (MRSA) infection including previous antibiotic use. J Antimicrob Chemother 2002; 49:99–105.

68. Weber SG, Gold HS, Hooper DC, et al. Fluoroquinolones and the risk for methicillin-resistant *Staphylococcus aureus* in hospitalized patients. Emerg Infect Dis 2003; 9:1415–1422.

69. Dziekan G, Hahn A, Thune K, et al. Methicillin-resistant *Staphylococcus aureus* in a teaching hospital: investigation of nosocomial transmission using a matched case-control study. J Hosp Infect 2000; 46:263–270.

70. Bergstrom CT, Lo M, Lipsitch M. Ecological theory suggests that antimicrobial cycling will not reduce antimicrobial resistance in hospitals. Proc Natl Acad Sci U S A 2004; 101:13285–13290.

71. Mori N, Hitomi S, Nakajima J, et al. Unselective use of intranasal mupirocin ointment for controlling propagation of methicillin-resistant *Staphylococcus aureus* in a thoracic surgery ward. J Infect Chemother 2005; 11:231–233.

72. Fawley WN, Parnel P, Hall J, et al. Surveillance for mupirocin resistance following introduction of routine perioperative prophylaxis with nasal mupirocin. J Hosp Infect 2006; 62:327–332.

73. Muller A, Talon D, Potier A, et al. Use of intranasal mupirocin to prevent methicillin-resistant *Staphylococcus aureus* infection in intensive care units. Crit Care Med 2005; 9:R246–R250.

74. Laupland KB, Conly JM. Treatment of *Staphylococcus aureus* colonization and prophylaxis for infection with topical intranasal mupirocin: an evidence-based review. Clin Infect Dis 2003; 37:933–938.

75. Hurdle JG, O'Neill AJ, Mody L, et al. In vivo transfer of high level mupirocin resistance from *Staphylococcus epidermidis* to methicillin-resistant

Staphylococus aureus associated with failure of mupirocin prophylaxis. J Antimicrob Chemother 2005; 56:1166–1168.

76. Cavdar C, Atay T, Zeybel M, et al. Emergence of resistance in staphylococci after long-term mupirocin application in patient on continuous ambulatory dialysis. Adv Perit Dial 2004; 20:67–70.

77. Schmitz FJ, Fluit AC, Hafner D, et al. Development of resistance to ciprofloxacin, rifampin and mupirocin in methicillin-susceptible and -resistant *Staphylococcus aureus* isolates. Antimicrob Agents Chemother 2000; 44:3229–3231.

78. Rupp ME, Lisco SJ, Lipsett PA, et al. Effect of a second-generation venous catheter impregnated with chlorhexidine and silver sulfadiazine on central catheter-related infections. Ann Intern Med 2005; 143:570–580.

79. Lubelchek RJ, Weinstein RA. Strategies for preventing catheter-related bloodstream infections: the role of new technologies. Crit Care Med 2006; 34:905–907.

80. O'Grady NP, Alexander M, Dellinger EP, et al. Guidelines for the prevention of intravascular catheter-related infections. MMWR 2002; 51(No. RR-10):1–36.

81. Widmer AF. Intravenous-related infections. In: Wenzel RP, ed. Prevention and Control of Nosocomial Infections. Philadelphia: Williams & Wilkins, 1997:771–805.

82. Rubinson L, Wu AW, Haponik EF, et al. Why is it that internist do not follow guidelines for preventing intravascular catheter infections? Infect Control Hosp Epidemiol 2005; 26:525–533.

83. Adams D, Quayum M, Worthington T, et al. Evaluation of a 2% chlorhexidine in 70 isopropyl alcohol skin disinfectant. J Hosp Infect 2005; 61:287–290.

84. Chaiyakunapruk N, Veenstra DL, Lipsky BA, et al. Chlorhexidine compared with povidone solution for vascular catheter site care: a meta analysis. Ann Intern Med 2002; 136:792–801.

85. Kollef MH, Shorr A, Tabak YP, et al. Epidemiology and outcome of healthcare-associated pneumonia: results from a large US database of culture positive pneumonia. Chest 2005; 128:3854–3862.

86. Rello J, Torres A, Ricart M, et al. Ventilator-associated pneumonia by *Staphylococcus aureus*. Am J Respir Crit Care Med 1994; 150:1545–1549.

87. Flanders SA, Collard HR, Saint S. Nosocomial pneumonia: state of the science. Am J Infect Control 2006; 54:84–93.

88. Tablan OC, Anderson LJ, Besser R, et al. Guidelines for preventing healthcare-associated pneumonia. MMWR 2004; 53(RR03):1–36.
89. Gaynes RP. Surveillance of nosocomial infections: a fundamental ingredient for quality. Infect Control Hosp Epidemiol 1997; 18:475–478.
90. National Nosocomial Infection Surveillance System. National Nosocomial Infections Surveillance (NNIS) System report, data summary from January 1992 through June 2004, issues October 2004. Am J Infect Control 2004; 32:470–485.
91. Wise LC, Hoffman J, Grant L, et al. Nursing wound care survey: sterile and nonsterile glove choice. J Wound Ostomy Continence Nurs 1997; 24:144–150.
92. Edward-Jones V. Antimicrobial and barrier effect of silver against methicillin-resistant *Staphylococcus aureus*. J Wound Care 2006; 15:285–290.
93. Strohal R, Schelling M, Takacs M, et al. Nanocrystalline silver dressing as an efficient anti-MRSA barrier: a new solution to an increasing problem. J Hosp Infect 2005; 60:226–230.
94. Mueller SW, Krebsbach LE. Impact of an antimicrobial-impregnated gauze dressing on surgical site infections including methicillin-resistant *Staphylococcus aureus*. Am J Infect Control 2008; 36:651–656.
95. Edmiston CE, Goheen MP, Krepel C, et al. Bacterial adherence to surgical sutures: is there a role for antibacterial-coated sutures in reducing the risk of surgical site infections? J Am Coll Surg 2006; 203:481–489.
96. Ford HR, Jones P, Gaines B, et al. Intraoperative handing and wound healing: controlled clinical trial comparing coated Vicryl Plus® suture. Surg Infect (Larchmt) 2005; 6:313–321.
97. Justinger C, Moussavian MR, Schlueter C, et al. Antibiotic coating of abdominal closure sutures and wound infection. Surgery 2009; 145:330–334.
98. Bratzler DW, Houck PM. Antimicrobial prophylaxis for surgery: an advisory statement from the National Surgical Infection Prevention project. Clin Infect Dis 2004; 38:1706–1715.
99. Edmiston CE, Krepel CJ, Seabrook GR, et al. The preoperative shower revisited: can high topical antiseptic levels be achieved on the skin surface prior to surgical admission? J Am Coll Surg 2008; 207:233–239.
100. Rosenstein AH. Hospital report cards: intent, impact and illusion. Am J Med Quality 2004; 19:183–192.
101. McKibben L, Fowler I, Horan T, et al. Ensuring rational public reporting systems for health care-associated infections: systematic literature review and evaluation recommendations. Am J Infect Control 2006; 34:142–149.

MRSA Prevention and Control

Renae E. Stafford
Division of Trauma and Critical Care Surgery, University of North Carolina
Department of Surgery

INTRODUCTION

Methicillin-resistant *Staphylococcus aureus* (MRSA) accounts for significant morbidity and mortality worldwide. In the United States, *S. aureus* has been isolated from 14.5% of all health care–associated infections (HAI) reported by acute care hospitals and other health care facilities to the National Healthcare Safety Network (NHSN) over a recent 22-month period (1). Over 50% of the staphylococcal infections that were device related and 49.2% of the surgical site infections (SSIs) had methicillin-resistant organisms isolated. Central line–associated bloodstream infections (CLABSI) are the most commonly reported HAIs. The overall proportion of *S. aureus* CLABSI in ICUs has increased between 1997 and 2007 by 25.8% (2). Similar data are reported in Europe where methicillin resistance was found between 2.2% and 92% of isolates from ICU *S. aureus* HAIs (3). Even higher resistance rates have been identified in a worldwide surveillance system (4).

There is an increased length of stay, mortality, and monetary health care costs associated with MRSA HAIs (5,6). This has led to increased efforts on national and international levels to prevent HAI and in particular to target the prevention and control of MRSA spread (7–13). Guidelines and consensus statements developed by multiple organizations have been published that address the prevention of antimicrobial resistance and also specifically target MRSA (14–18). This chapter will outline basic infection control strategies as well as specific strategies recommended to prevent and control spread of MRSA colonization and associated HAIs.

HAND HYGIENE

Patient-to-patient transmission of MRSA occurs primarily via transient colonization through the hands of the health care worker (15). Hand hygiene is an essential intervention to prevent the spread of health care–associated infections (7,19) and MRSA (20) and is promoted by the Institute for Healthcare Improvement as part of a "bundle" to reduce CLABSI (21). Hand hygiene is best implemented using soap and water and/or commercially available alcohol-based gels or foams. It should be performed upon entering a patient room, after patient contact (with or without gloves), moving from a contaminated to a clean body site, before and after inserting/manipulating invasive devices, and when leaving a patient room. While hand hygiene is a recognized cornerstone of infection control, rates of compliance documented in the literature are low and multiple approaches to increasing the compliance rates have been attempted. Multiple barriers exist to compliance with hand hygiene such as poor understanding of its importance, institutional lack of commitment, and unavailability of gels, foams, and sinks (22,23). Many interventions to increase compliance are directed at eliminating these barriers.

One large hospital system that encompasses nine facilities with between 22 and 950 beds was able to increase its hand hygiene compliance from 49% at baseline to 98% at the end of a multimodal intervention, and this increase in compliance was sustainable (24). Interventions included nursing and physician memos and poster boards, posters, hand hygiene fairs, buttons, internal marketing, and visitor education programs. A decrease in MRSA HAIs from 0.52 per 1000 patient days to 0.24 per 1000 patient days was documented.

Behavioral approaches for handwashing include direct monitoring and feedback of data to health care workers (25,26), culture change using positive deviance technique (8), and education programs including participatory decision making (10). Direct monitoring and feedback of data was associated with a decrease in facility-acquired MRSA from 0.85 per

1000 patient days to 0.52 per 1000 patient days one year after the intervention (25). The investigators note that this represents 51 avoided infections at a potential savings of between $1,020,000 and $1,785,000. Feedback on infection control practices and ward-acquired MRSA rates using statistical process control charts showed a statistically significant and sustained decrease in MRSA rates (26). Mandatory education programs decrease the rates of nosocomial acquisition of MRSA colonization or infection; however, this intervention is usually not sufficient to increase hand hygiene compliance (10).

ENVIRONMENTAL HYGIENE

Since hand hygiene is important for preventing transmission of MRSA, it is logical that the health care environment should also be clean. Contact with contaminated equipment and surfaces is implicated in MRSA spread (7,20). One would hypothesize that enhanced cleaning of inanimate objects and surfaces in the health care environment would decrease transmission. Collaboration with environmental management in health care facilities is often a part of a multidisciplinary approach to decreasing nosocomial transmission of MRSA (8,14,15,20) and other HAIs (7,27,28).

Recommendations for environmental hygiene include protocols for cleaning and disinfecting environmental surfaces using appropriate agents, for daily and terminal cleaning of patient rooms, for "high touch" surfaces such as bed rails and doorknobs, and for cleaning and disinfecting patient care equipment (20). It is also recommended to dedicate noncritical patient care items such as blood pressure cuffs and stethoscopes to known colonized or infected patients. MRSA-contaminated stethoscopes can be adequately disinfected with 70% alcohol swabs or other hospital disinfectants (20,29).

Cleaning regimens using detergent and 1% hypochlorite solution on patient-specific sites touched by health care workers such as ventilators and infusion pumps, those touched by health care worker and visitors such as the bedside stand, and other sites such as computer keypads are effective in removing MRSA from the immediate environment; however, postcleaning recontamination was observed in a seven-hour surveillance period after the cleaning (30). This study documents that recontamination occurred primarily at sites touched by health care workers. This suggests a break in infection control practices such as handwashing.

Another study using an enhanced cleaning regimen with extra personnel compared to the standard cleaning regimen in a prospective crossover study method showed a measurable effect on the clinical environment (31). Aerobic colony counts were reduced by 32.5% overall; however, no difference in recovery of MRSA was seen. Despite this, there was a decrease in the number of new MRSA infections seen although the study was not well powered to detect true differences. Unfortunately, a rebound effect was seen after withdrawal of the enhanced cleaning.

Despite the lack of specific evidence for a decrease in nosocomial transmission of MRSA, it stands to reason that basic environmental hygiene is an important component of any infection control program (15). Current data suggest that environmental hygiene alone is not sufficient to prevent transmission of MRSA and other HAIs.

PATIENT HYGIENE

While health care workers are thought to be the primary agent for nosocomial patient-to-patient transmission of MRSA, it is the colonized or infected patient who serves as the MRSA reservoir. Decreasing colonization of the patient would decrease the available pool of patients, serving as a reservoir for transmission. Historically, the emphasis has been placed on patients already in the hospital. The emergence of community-acquired MRSA (CA-MRSA), which is genotypically different than health care–associated MRSA (HC-MRSA), has led to limited efforts to break the cycle of transmission and spread of MRSA in the community (11). These patients contact the health care system as an outpatient and an inpatient. Thus, CA-MRSA reservoirs now exist in the hospital and are transmitted via the same vectors as HC-MRSA (32). Additionally, patients who are discharged with HC-MRSA to long-term care settings and nursing homes serve as community reservoirs for HC-MRSA spread outside the hospital. The ubiquitous nature of MRSA in our health care facilities and community suggest that routine patient hygiene in compliance with infection control principles for the hospital may need to become commonplace in the community.

Recent studies suggest that daily chlorhexidine bathing of patients in an ICU can decrease VRE bacteremia (33). MRSA acquisition was reduced by 32%, but there was no difference in rates of MRSA bacteremia. This is likely because of the low baseline incidence of MRSA bacteremia (34). Single interventions are not effective because of breaks in technique for infection control practices, but daily chlorhexidine baths are warranted as an additional tool in a multipronged approach to decreasing transmission.

DECOLONIZATION

Colonization pressure has a significant effect on transmission of MRSA (35). Decolonization of known carriers of MRSA (colonized or infected) is proposed as a means to decrease the colonization pressure and subsequent transmission (36). However, decolonization of patients and health care workers is a subject of great debate. The issues include cost of identification and treatment of carriers, resource utilization, and the development of resistance to agents used for decolonization and effectiveness and side effects of the treatment.

S. aureus carriers are primarily colonized in the anterior nares, but other sites of carriage include surgical wounds, decubitus ulcers, and medical device sites (36,37). While most infections are the result of endogenous source, exogenous sources such as health care workers and other patients are also potential sources. Decolonization treatments, therefore, focus primarily on therapy applied to the anterior nares and, on some occasions, topical therapy to the skin.

Multiple agents can eradicate nasal carriage of *S. aureus* (MSSA and MRSA) in both topical and systemic form either alone or in combination (36,37). The most extensively studied agent is topical 2% mupirocin ointment that is efficacious for nasal decolonization but is less effective for extranasal sites. This agent is the only FDA-approved topical agent for eradication of MRSA nasal colonization in adults. This agent requires a prescription and is active against most gram-positive and gram-negative bacteria including MSSA, MRSA, and coagulase-negative staphylococci. Adverse events typically include headache, rhinitis, and congestion and stinging at the application site. Two recent studies show conflicting results when studying the application of mupirocin to the nares of patients who screened positive for MRSA (38,39). The studies differed in their approaches to screening, monitoring, and therapeutic compliance, making the data difficult to interpret. Other topical applications to the anterior nares include bacitracin ointment, neomycin/triple antibiotic ointment, tea tree oil, and retapamulin (37). These agents have been studied in an attempt to find an alternative when mupirocin resistance develops.

The exact dosing and number of applications needed to be effective is not clear (40). In addition, the ability to provide long-term eradication is not clear. Because of the difficulty in eradicating *S. aureus* from extranasal sites, a combination of topical and systemic therapy may be warranted. Other agents have been identified as potential therapies and are beyond the scope of this discussion. A detailed review can be found in the Simor (36) and McConeghy (37).

Given known limitations of decolonization therapy, there are no blanket recommendations for decolonization therapy for MRSA-colonized patients or health care workers. However, certain patients may benefit from therapy as well as health care workers identified as possible vectors during an outbreak of MRSA infections in the health care setting. Outbreaks of MRSA may occur in the community with ongoing transmission in cohorts such as households, sports teams, and nursing facilities. Contact tracing and decolonization in this setting may interrupt further transmission. Recommendations for selective decontamination of selected patient and health care worker populations are available from a number of organizations (14,15,20).

Nasal carriage of MRSA is a risk factor for subsequent infection in surgical patients, and such patients are of particular interest for decolonization. SSIs are the third most common type of HAI with *S. aureus* being the second most common pathogen behind coagulase-negative *Staphylococcus* (1). 49.2% of those SSIs caused by *S. aureus* are methicillin resistant. SSIs are associated with increased duration of hospital stay, cost, morbidity, and mortality (41). Certain subgroups of patients are at particular risk for carriage of MRSA and subsequent SSI. Cardiothoracic surgery and vascular patients are often found to be carriers with increased risk of infection (42). MRSA colonization in vascular patients was related to subsequent infection with an odds ratio of 65 (43). Other studies show similar relationships in surgical patients admitted on an emergency basis (44). SSI prevention interventions for MRSA are probably cost effective and achievable. (45,46).

Decolonization of health care workers can be a potentially contentious topic. Most workers are transient carriers of MRSA. Whether or not health care workers who are identified as being carriers should be removed from clinical care duties and made to undergo decolonization with topical mupirocin is not clear. The endemicity of the organism and different screening strategies in various hospitals and countries will aid in the determination of an appropriate strategy (15). It may be useful in outbreak situations where health care workers are identified as potential reservoirs and are at risk themselves for the development of serious infections (11,47).

LABORATORY SCREENING AND SURVEILLANCE FOR COLONIZATION AND INFECTION

Screening and surveillance programs for MRSA colonization and infection are well described, but there are no clear recommendations for screening all patients in an active manner. Screening may be done either alone or in combination with other infection control practices such as decolonization, cohorting, and isolation of patients found to be carriers of MRSA. These programs can screen all patients or only a selected patient population. Active screening involves the systematic use of microbiologic tests that are able to detect mucocutaneous carriage of MRSA by individuals without active infection (13).

Screening for colonization is done by a number of methods. Swabbing of the anterior nares is the most common method used. Nasal screening has a sensitivity of over 80% (13). Conventional methods rely on selective culture on media and results may not be available for up to 72 hours. More rapid methods using PCR techniques are available and can lead to earlier detection and isolation of carriers.

Random screening and surveillance along with systematic decolonization of identified carriers reduces the carriage rate and the pool of MRSA carriers (12). In a selected group of surgical patients in a Surgical Infection Prevention Project, active surveillance and decolonization of carriers with 2% nasal mupirocin two times a day for five days and alternate day chlorhexidine baths reduced the rate of MRSA SSI (48). Others have shown a benefit to universal surveillance (38) but other studies contradict this approach (39).

Patients in intensive care units are a particular population of interest. In a review of the available literature on active screening of adult patients in intensive care units, no definitive recommendation could be made (49). In one study where no active surveillance for MRSA was done in the ICU and other multiple evidence-based infection control practices were carried out, there was a reduction in all infections including those caused by MRSA (50).

There is no clear consensus with respect to what all of the components of an active surveillance program are—who should be screened, when and how often should patients be screened, and should those identified as carriers all be decolonized? Some authors argue that screening for MRSA is a flawed hospital infection control intervention (51). An approach to the control of MRSA without a broader infection control program would fail as many other drug-resistant pathogens are becoming more prevalent. The argument suggests a population-based intervention targeting all drug-resistant pathogens.

Current recommendations with respect to screening and surveillance include that it should be driven by need (13). A screening example would be screening patients with risk factors for colonization who are in high-risk patient care areas (13,27). A surveillance example would be active surveillance cultures of all high-risk patients (16). Any screening and surveillance program should be part of a multifaceted strategy to prevent transmission when there is ongoing transmission of MRSA despite effective implementation of basic infection control practices (20).

The criteria for screening of health care workers for MRSA colonization or infection, like the recommendations for decolonization, are that they be tested only if they are linked to a cluster or outbreak of MRSA or are working in areas of low endemicity (11,15,20).

ANTIBIOTIC STEWARDSHIP

High antibiotic exposure is a documented risk factor for the development of HC-MRSA and is particularly important in the development of CA-MRSA (52). Reducing the inappropriate use of antibiotics promotes the concept of antibiotic stewardship (53). A successful antibiotic stewardship program includes the same behavioral techniques used to improve compliance with hand hygiene. Auditing of antibiotic use, reporting and feedback of data regarding antibiotic use and MRSA prevalence to appropriate clinicians and health care workers, automatic discontinuation of perioperative antibiotics in appropriate surgical patients, and discontinuation of empiric therapy with negative cultures all may prove to be effective as part of a multifaceted approach to limit antibiotic pressure in the health care setting (53,54). Other interventions, such as formulary restriction and preauthorization for the use of certain antibiotics and postprescription review of antibiotic, are recommended (54,55). In one institution where both a "front end" and "back end" approach were used as part of an antibiotic stewardship program, there was a decrease in the total consumption of antibiotics, and a stabilization in the trend toward increasing resistance without an increase in patient mortality. Recommendations are that antibiotic stewardship should be part of a comprehensive infection control program (56) and should apply to all practitioners (55).

ISOLATION PRACTICES

Isolation of patients who are at risk for transmission of MRSA or infected with MRSA, along with hand hygiene, is a basic foundation of control of spread of infection (15,16,20). However, when and how to isolate these patients varies depending on hospital infection control strategies and is not without risk. Placing patients into isolation is associated with increased risk of adverse events, less patient contact, and development of decubitus ulcers and may have psychological effects (20). Isolation or cohorting may be done in a number of ways. If the hospital protocols mandate screening of all high-risk patients, those patients may actually be placed in a private room and on isolation precautions until their screening tests are negative and continued on them if positive. This is an expensive fiscal proposition for any institution.

Placing patients on isolation is done by placing them in a single room or as part of a cohort unit (in a room with another positive patient). However, in a given institution, the ability to adequately isolate patients will depend on available resources and may lead to the need to triage those patients at greatest risk for transmission to the top of the list for available rooms (15). One novel approach where patients were cohorted in a dedicated unit reduced hospital-acquired methicillin-resistant *S. aureus* infection (57). Patient benefits included freedom to ambulate throughout the unit and decreased levels of visitor and patient emotional stress. Other ancillary benefits included a decrease in expenditures for isolation gowns, decreased length of stay, and a hand hygiene compliance of over 90%. This type of cohorting actually decreases the colonization pressure in the remainder of the hospital. A similar approach, but in reverse, was done by creating an orthopedic surgery unit specifically for admission of patients with a recent negative MRSA screen (58).

In addition to physically isolating patients, they are at a minimum put on contact precautions. This requires that all health care workers who come into contact with the patient wear gowns and gloves in addition to standard protocols whenever they enter a patient room (20). Hospitals must also have a defined policy for discontinuation of isolation and contact precautions. Because colonization can last months, in the absence of specific decolonization protocols, contact precautions are recommended throughout the hospital stay.

CONCLUSION

There are many effective methods for prevention and control of transmission of infection with MRSA. Given the fact that multiple strategies are often used simultaneously as part of a comprehensive infection control strategy, no one intervention can be singled out as being the most effective or important. Clearly, broadly based strategies that include antibiotic stewardship, hand hygiene compliance, patient hygiene, environmental hygiene, and isolation and cohorting of patients colonized or infected with multidrug-resistant (MDR) organisms will affect not only MRSA prevention and transmission but also transmission of other MDR organisms. All institutions should have fully developed and implemented infection control practices targeted against the prevention of health care–associated infections in general (7,17,18). Interventions more specifically related to MRSA prevention such as active surveillance, preemptive isolation, and cohorting and decolonization are also effective. However, their effectiveness will vary on whether MRSA is endemic, whether resources are available for testing, treatment and isolation, and on the compliance with and reliability of the screening and decolonization. Guidelines for their use are well defined (14,15,20,27). These interventions should be used as adjuncts to basic infection control strategies. More novel approaches to MRSA prevention and control based on the structure of hospital social networks (59) and industrial systems engineering (9) may continue to be proven useful with future study and implementation.

REFERENCES

1. Hidron AI, Edwards JR, Patel J, et al. Antimicrobial resistant pathogens associated with healthcare-associated infections: annual summary of data reported to the National healthcare Safety network at the Centers for Disease Control and Prevention, 2006–2007. Infect Control Hosp Epidemiol 2008; 29:996–1011.
2. Burton DC, Edwards JR, Horan TC, et al. Methicillin-resistant *Staphylococcus aureus* central line-associated bloodstream infections in US intensive care units, 1997–2007. JAMA 2009; 727–736.
3. Hanberger H, Arman D, Gill H, et al. Surveillance of microbial resistance in European intensive care units: a first report from the Care-ICU programme for improved infection control. Intensive Care Med 2009; 35:91–100.
4. Rosenthal VD, Maki DG, Mehta A, et al. International nosocomial infection control consortium report, data summary for 2002–2007, issued January 2008. Am J Infect Control 2008; 36:627–637.
5. Cosgrove SE, Sakoulas G, Perencevich EN, et al. Comparison of mortality associated with methicillin-resistant and methicillin-susceptible *Staphylococcus aureus* bacteremia: a meta-analysis. Clin Infect Dis 2003; 36:53–59.
6. Cosgrove SE, Qi Y, Kaye KS, et al. The impact of methicillin-resistant *Staphylococcus aureus* bacteremia on patient outcomes: mortality, length of stay, and hospital charges. Infect Control Hosp Epidemiol 2005; 26:166–174.
7. Doshi RK, Patel G, MacKay R, et al. Healthcare-associated infections: Epidemiology, prevention and therapy. Mount Sinai J Med 2009; 76:84–94.

8. Bonuel N, Byers P, Gray-Becknell T. Methicillin resistant *Staphylococcus aureus* (MRSA) prevention through facility-wide culture change. Crit Care Nurs Q 2009; 32:144–148.

9. Muder RR, Cunningham CC, McCray E, et al. Implementation of an industrial systems engineering approach to reduce the incidence of methicillin-resistant *Staphylococcus aureus* infection. Infect Control Hosp Epidemiol 2008; 29:702–708.

10. Lee TC, Moore C, Raboud JM, et al. Impact of a mandatory infection control education program on nosocomial acquisition of methicillin-resistant *Staphylococcus aureus*. Infect Control Hosp Epidemiol 2009; 30:249–256.

11. Navarro M, Huttner B, Harbarth S. Methicillin-resistant *Staphylococcus aureus* control in the 21st century: beyond the acute care hospital. Curr Opin Infect Dis 2008; 21:372–379.

12. Karas JA, Enoch DA, Eagle HJ, et al. Random methicillin-resistant *Staphylococcus aureus* carrier surveillance at a district hospital and the impact of interventions to reduce endemic carriage. J Hosp Infect 2009; 71:327–332.

13. Struelens MJ, Hawkey PM, French GL, et al. Laboratory tools and strategies for methicillin-resistant *Staphylococcus aureus* screening, surveillance and typing: state of the art and unmet needs. Clin Microbiol Infect 2009; 15:112–119.

14. Gould FK, Brindle R, Chadwick PR, et al. Guidelines (2008) for the prophylaxis and treatment of methicillin-resistant *Staphylococcus aureus* (MRSA) infections in the United Kingdom. J Antimicrob Chemother 2009; 63:849–861.

15. Humphreys H, Grundmann H, Skov R, et al. Prevention and control of methicillin-resistant *Staphylococcus aureus*. Clin Microb Infect 2009; 15:120–124.

16. Muto CA, Jernigan JA, Ostrowsky BE, et al. SHEA guideline for preventing nosocomial transmission of multidrug-resistant strains of *Staphylococcus aureus* and *Enterococcus*. Infect Control Hosp Epidemiol 2003; 24:362–386.

17. Mackenzie FM, Struelens MJ, Towener KJ, et al. On behalf of the ARPAC Steering Group and the ARPAC Consensus Conference Participants. Report of the Consensus Conference on antibiotic resistance, prevention and control (ARPAC). Clin Microbiol Infect 2005; 11:937–954.

18. Shlaes DM, Gerding DN, John JF, et al. Society for Healthcare Epidemiology of America and Infectious Disease Society of America Joint Committee on the Prevention of Antimicrobial resistance: guidelines for the prevention of antimicrobial resistance in hospitals. Infect Control Hosp Epidemiol 1997; 18:275–291.

19. Boyce JM, Pittet D; Healthcare Infection Control Practices Advisory Committee; HICPAC/SHEA/APICIDSA Hand Hygiene Task Force. Guidelines for hand hygiene in health-care settings. MMWR Recomm Rep 2002; 51(RR-16):1–45.

20. Calfee DP, Salgado CD, Classen D, et al. Strategies to prevent transmission of methicillin-resistant *Staphylococcus aureus* in acute care hospitals. SHEA/IDSA Practice Recommendation. Infect Control Hosp Epidemiol 2008; 29: S62–S80.

21. Institute for Healthcare Improvement. Implement the central line bundle. Available at: www.ihi.org/ihi/topics/criticalcare/intensivecare/changes/implementthecentrallinebundle.htm. Accessed August 8, 2009.

22. Centers for Disease Control and Prevention. Hand hygiene core slides. Available at: www.cdc.gov/handhygiene/download/hand_hygiene_core.ppt. Accessed August 8, 2009.

23. Institute for Healthcare Improvement. How-to guide. Getting started kit: prevent central line infections. Available at: www.ihi.org/ihi/programs/Campaign. Accessed August 8, 2009.

24. Lederer JW, Best D, Hendrix V. A comprehensive hygiene approach to reducing MRSA health care-associated infections. J Joint Commission Qual Patient Safety 2009; 35:180–185.

25. Cromer AL, Latham SC, Bryant KG, et al. Monitoring and feedback of hand hygiene compliance and the impact on facility-acquired methicillin-resistant *Staphylococcus aureus*. Am J Infect Control 2008; 36:672–677.

26. Curran E, Harper P, Loveday H, et al. Results of a multicentre randomised controlled trial of statistical process control charts and structured diagnostic tools to reduce ward-acquired methicillin-resistant *Staphylococcus aureus*: the CHART project. J Hosp Infect 2008; 70:127–135.

27. Johnston BL, Bryce E. Hospital infection control strategies for vancomycin-resistant *Enterococcus*, methicillin-resistant *Staphylococcus aureus* and *Clostridium difficile*. CMA J 2009; 180:627–631.

28. Mears A, White A, Cookson B, et al. Healthcare-associated infection in acute hospitals: which interventions are effective? J Hosp Infect 2009; 71:307–313.

29. Fenelon L, Holcroft L, Waters N. Contamination of stethoscopes with MRSA and current disinfection practices. J Hosp Infect 2009; 376–378.

30. Aldeyab M, McElnay JC, Elshibly SM, et al. Evaluation of the efficacy of a conventional cleaning regimen in removing methicillin-resistant *Staphylococcus aureus* from contaminated surfaces in an intensive care unit. Infect Control Hosp Epidemiol 2009; 30:304–305.

31. Dancer SJ, White LF, Lamb J, et al. Measuring the effect of enhanced cleaning in a UK hospital: a prospective crossover study. BMC Med 2009; 7:28.

32. Reygaert W. Methicillin-resistant *Staphylococcus aureus* (MRSA): Prevalence and epidemiology issues. Clin Lab Sci 2009; 22:111–114.

33. Climo MW, Sepkowitz KA, Zuccotti G, et al. The effect of daily bathing with chlorhexidine on the acquisition of methicillin-resistant *Staphylococcus aureus*, vancomycin-resistant *Enterococcus,* and healthcare-associated infections: Results of a quasi-experimental multicenter trial. Crit Care Med 2009; 37:1858–1865.

34. Parienti JJ. A paradigm shift to prevent nosocomial infection: "Take a bath before I touch you." Crit Care Med 2009; 37:2097–2098.

35. Williams VR, Callery S, Vearncombe M, et al. The role of colonization pressure in nosocomial transmission of methicillin-resistant *Staphylococcus aureus*. Am J Infect Control 2009; 37:106–110.

36. Simor AE, Danerman N. *Staphylococcus aureus* decolonization as a prevention strategy. Infect Dis Clin N Am 2009; 23:133–151.

37. McConeghy KW, Mickolich DJ, LaPlante KL. Agents for the decolonization of methicillin-resistant *Staphylococcus aureus*. Pharmacotherapy 2009; 29:263–280.

38. Robicsek A, Beaumont JL, Paule SM, et al. Universal surveillance for methicillin-resistant *Staphylococcus aureus* in 3 affiliated hospitals. Ann Intern Med 2008; 148:409–418.

39. Harbarth S, Fankhauser C, Schrenzel J, et al. Universal screening for methicillin-resistant *Staphylococcus aureus* at hospital admission and nosocomial infections in surgical patients. JAMA 2008; 299:1149–1157.

40. Cavdar C, Saglam F, Sifil A, et al. Effect of once-a-week vs. thrice-a-week application of mupirocin on methicillin and mupirocin resistance in peritoneal dialysis patients: three years of experience. Renal Failure 2008; 30:417–422.

41. Anderson DJ, Kaye KS. Staphylococcal surgical site infections. Infect Dis Clin N Am 2009; 23:53–72.

42. Munoz P, Hortal J, Gianella M, et al. Nasal carriage of *S. aureus* increases the risk of surgical site infection after major heart surgery. J Hosp Infect 2008; 68:25–31.

43. Morange-Saussier V, Giraudeau B, van der Mee N, et al. Nasal carriage of methicillin-resistant *Staphylococcus aureus* in vascular surgery. Ann Vasc Surg 2006; 20:767–772.

44. Muralidhar B, Anwar SM, Handa A, et al. Prevalence of MRSA in emergency and elective patients admitted to a vascular surgical unit: implications of antibiotic prophylaxis. Eur J Vasc Endovasc Surg 2006; 32:402–407.

45. van Rijen M, Kluytmans J. New approaches to prevention of staphylococcal infection in surgery. Curr Opin Infect Dis 2008; 21:380–384.

46. Anderson DJ, Chen LF, Schmader KE, et al. Poor functional status as a risk factor for surgical site infection due to methicillin-resistant *Staphylococcus aureus*. Infect Control Hosp Epidemiol 2008; 29:832–839.

47. Khan A, Lampitoc M, Salaripour M, et al. Rapid control of a methicillin resistant *Staphylococcus aureus* (MRSA) outbreak in a medical surgical intensive care unit (ICU). Can J Infect Control 2009; 24(1):12–16.

48. Pofahl WE, Goettler CE, Ramsey KM, et al. Active surveillance screening of MRSA and eradication of the carrier state decreases surgical-site infections caused by MRSA. J Am Coll Surg 2009; 208(5):981–986.

49. McGinigle KL, Gourley ML, Buchanan IB. The use of active surveillance cultures in adults in intensive care units to reduce methicillin-resistant *Staphylococcus aureus*–related morbidity, mortality and costs: a systematic review. Clin Infect Dis 2008; 46:1717–1725.

50. Edmond MB, Ober JF, Bearman G. Active surveillance cultures are not required to control MRSA infections in the critical care setting. Am J Infect Control 2008; 36:461–463.

51. Wenzel RP, Bearman G, Edmond M. Screening for MRSA: a flawed hospital infection control intervention. Infect Control Hosp Epidemiol 2008; 29: 1012–1018.

52. Gould IM. Antibiotics, skin and soft tissue infection and methicillin-resistant *Staphylococcus aureus*: cause and effect. Int J Antimicrob Agents 2009; S8–S11.

53. Septimus EJ, Kuper KM. Clinical challenges in addressing resistance to antimicrobial drugs in the twenty-first century. Clin Pharmacol Ther 2009; 86(3):336–339.

54. Dellit TH, Owens RC, McGowan JE, et al. Infectious Disease Society and the Society for Healthcare Epidemiology of America guidelines for developing an institutional program to enhance antimicrobial stewardship. Clin Infect Dis 2007; 44:159–177.

55. Santos RP, Magedanz L, Siliprandi E. Antimicrobial stewardship programs must apply to all. Infect Control Hosp Epidemiol 2009; 30:205–207.

56. Brinsley K, Sinkowitz-Cochran R, Cardo D, et al. CDC campaign to prevent antimicrobial resistance team. An assessment of issues surrounding

implementation of the campaign to prevent resistance in healthcare settings. Am J Infect Control 2005; 33:402–409.

57. Gilroy SA, Stahl BM, Noona C, et al. Reduction of hospital-acquired methicillin-resistant *Staphylococcus aureus* infection by cohorting patients in a dedicated unit. Infect Control Hosp Epidemiol 2009; 30:203–205.

58. Biant LC, Teare EL, Williams WW, et al. Eradication of methicillin-resistant *Staphylococcus aureus* by "ring fencing" of elective orthopedic beds. Br Med J 2004; 329:149–151.

59. Ueno T, Masuda N. Controlling nosocomial infection based on structure of hospital social networks. J Theor Biol 2008; 254:655–666.

Outcomes and Cost Considerations with MRSA Infections

14

Jack E. Brown
State University of New York at Buffalo, Buffalo, New York, U.S.A.

Jeremy Dengler and Thomas P. Lodise, Jr.
Albany College of Pharmacy and Health Sciences, Albany, New York, U.S.A.

INTRODUCTION

Over the past two decades, rates of antimicrobial resistance have increased rapidly. Of the two million annual nosocomial infections in the United States, more than 50% are caused by drug-resistant strains of bacteria (1,2). Drug resistance has a considerable impact on patient morbidity and mortality, and is a major economic burden for society with yearly expenditures ranging from US$4 billion to US$30 billion (1–3).

One resistant organism of particular concern is methicillin-resistant *Staphylococcus aureus* (MRSA), which is endemic in many hospitals throughout the world (4–9). MRSA rates have been steadily climbing in both the intensive care unit (ICU) and non-ICU hospital setting. Among U.S. hospitals, MRSA is the most commonly isolated antibiotic-resistant pathogen, and accounts for more than half of all *S. aureus* isolates in many institutions (7,9); in domestic ICUs, the MRSA rate exceeds 70% (7–9).

Historically, MRSA infections have occurred primarily among hospitalized patients or among those with a history of extensive hospitalization and other predisposing risk factors such as indwelling catheters, past antimicrobial use, decubitis ulcers, a postoperative surgical wound, or treatment with enteral feedings or dialysis (10–26). There is, however, growing evidence suggesting that the epidemiology of MRSA is evolving: the drug-resistant strain is no longer exclusively confined to hospitals or limited to patients with traditional predisposing risk factors (27–45). Increasingly, reports document nascent community-associated MRSA (CA-MRSA) infection among healthy individuals without known risk factors for MRSA. Outbreaks of CA-MRSA are reported in men who have sex with men and in close-contact settings, such as prisons, child care centers, sports teams, and Native American Indian communities (27–39). CA-MRSA is endemic in certain areas and >10% of patients without a history of hospitalization in the preceding year that present to the hospital with an *S. aureus* infection are culture-positive for CA-MRSA (27,29,40,43–45). No longer limited to the community setting, a growing number of hospitals in the United States have reported that CA-MRSA strains are replacing health care–acquired MRSA (HC-MRSA) isolates as the predominant cause of MRSA infection in their institutions (44–46).

RELATIONSHIP BETWEEN MRSA AND OUTCOMES

MRSA and Mortality: Bloodstream Infections

In addition to the rising rates of MRSA in both the health care and community settings, concerns have been raised over the deleterious outcomes associated with MRSA infections, particularly MRSA bloodstream infections (BSIs) (15,47). Although contemporary mortality rates are much lower than the pre-antibiotic era, there has been a steady rise in *S. aureus* BSI (SA-BSI) case-fatality rates (5), and the current mortality rate is reported to be 15% to 60% (10,12,13,15–17,19,20,22,23,25,26, 48–54). Inspection of these studies shows that the death rate is usually higher among patients with MRSA BSI than patients with methicillin-susceptible *S. aureus* (MSSA) BSI.

Despite the higher crude mortality rates observed with MRSA BSI, its role in patient survival has been a contentious issue (10,12,13, 15–17,19,20,22,23,25,26,48–53). Many believe that the association between MRSA and patient outcomes can be explained by factors other than drug resistance. These confounding patient factors may independently contribute to adverse clinical outcomes.

Cosgrove et al. performed a meta-analysis to compare mortality rates among patients with BSI caused by MRSA and MSSA (15). These authors reviewed studies reporting mortality rates associated with both MRSA and MSSA BSIs from January 1980 through December 2000. Thirty-one cohort studies were identified with a total of 3963 SA-BSI patients. The etiology of the BSI was MSSA for 2603 (65.7%) patients and MRSA for 1360 (34.3%) patients. The pooled analysis revealed a statistically significant increase in mortality among patients with MRSA bacteremia [36.4% vs. 23.4%, respectively, $p < 0.01$, and pooled odds ratio (OR) of 1.93; 95% confidence interval (CI), 1.54–2.42; $p < 0.001$]. Cosgrove et al. tried to overcome the inherent heterogeneity among the studies by creating homogenous subgroups of studies, including a cohort of studies that controlled for disease severity. In all of these subgroup analyses, the OR between MRSA and death consistently remained at 1.56 to 2.2 and the association between MRSA and mortality persisted even when adjustments were made for severity of illness. On the basis of their findings, the authors cited type II error as the primary reason for heterogeneity among results of previous studies (15).

Whitby et al. performed a similar meta-analysis but limited the analysis to nosocomial BSI caused by *S. aureus* (53). They identified nine studies comprising 2209 nosocomial SA-BSI cases. All but one study found a significant relationship between MRSA and death with the relative risk of death being significantly higher for patients with BSI because of MRSA (29%) than MSSA (12%) (OR, 2.12; 95% CI, 1.76–2.57; $p < 0.001$) (53). These meta-analyses support the notion that the mortality difference between MRSA and MSSA is real, even after adjustment for severity of illness and comorbid conditions.

MRSA and Mortality: Ventilator-Associated Pneumonia

There have been a number of studies that have examined the relationship between MRSA and mortality among patients with ventilator-associated pneumonia (VAP) (55). Athanassa et al. performed a systematic literature review that included eight original research articles (55). They found that the crude in-hospital mortality was higher in patients with VAP because of MRSA than in those with VAP because of MSSA (OR, 1.79; 95% CI, 1.210–2.65). Only four of the eight studies considered disease severity and adequacy of treatment that might influence mortality in the multivariate analysis. After adjusting for these potential confounders, only one study found MRSA to be associated with mortality. Collectively, these studies suggest that patients with MRSA VAP have higher mortality rates relative to MSSA VAP and underscore the importance of adjusting for severity of illness and comorbid conditions.

MRSA and Morbidity

Despite the ongoing debate about the impact of MRSA on mortality, there is no doubt that MRSA treatment is costly, primarily because of the lengthy hospital stay and the professional costs incurred during admission (Table 1) (10,18,22,48,50,52,54,56–60). This is exemplified in a study conducted by Rubin et al. who reviewed hospital discharge data from the New York City metropolitan area in 1995 and estimated the incidence, death rate, and cost of *S. aureus* infection (52). During the single year of the study, 13,550 discharged patients had *S. aureus* infections, and 2780 (20.5%) of these were MRSA. The attributable cost of community-acquired MRSA was US$34,000 compared to US$31,500 for a patient with community-acquired MSSA. For nosocomial infections, the attributable cost of MRSA was US$31,400 compared to US$27,700 for MSSA (52).

TABLE 1 Comparison of Hospital Costs and Charges for MRSA and MSSA

Study	Population	Endpoint	MRSA (USD)	MSSA (USD)
Abramson et al. (7)	Nosocomial BSI	Median total cost of hospitalization attributable to BSI	27,083	9,661
Capitano et al. (46)	Infections in long-term care facility	Median infection cost	2,607	1,332
Cosgrove et al. (50)	Nosocomial BSI	Median hospital charges after onset of BSI	26,212	19,212
Engemann et al. (54)	Surgical site infections	Median hospital charges attributable to SSI	92,363	52,791
Lodise et al. (52)	Nosocomial BSI	Adjust mean cost after onset of BSI	21,577	11,668
McHugh et al. (48)	Nosocomial BSI	Mean cost per patient-day of hospitalization	5,878	2,073
Reed et al. (54)	BSI in dialysis patients	Adjusted mean cost of initial hospitalization	21,251	13,978
		Adjusted mean cost 12 weeks after initial hospitalization	25,518	17,354
Rubin et al. (50)	All infections	Attributable mean cost	34,000	31,500
	Nosocomial infections	Attributable mean cost	31,400	27,700
Wakefield et al. (53)	Nosocomial infections	Mean total cost of hospitalization directly attributable to infection	7,481	2,377
Ben-David et al.	ICU patients with BSI	Unadjusted median hospitalization costs	51,492	17,603

MRSA, methicillin-resistant *Staphylococcus aureus*; MSSA, methicillin-susceptible *S. aureus*; BSI, bloodstream infection.

These findings have been echoed by multiple other investigators who examined the impact of MRSA in the hospital setting (10,18,22,48,50,54,56–58). Shorr et al. found that patients with MRSA as compared to MSSA VAP had on average four days longer mechanical ventilation, five additional days of ICU time, and an additional US$7700 (60). In a study of 348 cases of SA-BSI (96 cases of MRSA) by Cosgrove et al., both the median length of hospitalization and median hospital charges after onset of SA-BSI were significantly increased among MRSA patients versus MSSA patients (9 vs. 7 days, $p < 0.05$; US$26,212 vs. US$19,212, $p = 0.008$) and these differences persisted following correction for baseline variables [1.29-fold increase in length of stay (LOS); $p = 0.016$; 1.36-fold increase in hospital charges; $p = 0.017$] (50). McHugh et al. reported higher costs among MRSA BSI than MSSA BSI. In this study, mean cost per patient-day of hospitalization was US$3805 higher for MRSA BSI than for MSSA BSI (US$5878 vs. US$2073; $p = 0.003$). When patients were stratified by their case mix index, a difference of US$5302 per patient-day was found between the two groups for all patients with a case mix index greater than 2 ($p < 0.001$) (22). These results were comparable to the study by Wakefield et al., which reported a US$5000 cost difference between MRSA and MSSA hospitalized infections (56). These cost differences are lower than the median attributable total cost difference reported by Abramson in a case-control study. The median cost difference between treating an MRSA BSI and an MSSA BSI was US$17,422 per patient (10). Lodise et al. also noted a stark contrast in LOS and hospitalization costs between MRSA and MSSA bacteremic patients. After adjusting for confounding variables, MRSA bacteremia was associated with a 1.5-fold longer LOS (19.1 days vs. 14.2 days, $p = 0.005$) and a twofold increase in adjusted mean hospitalization costs (US$21,577 vs. US$11,668, $p = 0.001$) (54). In another case-control study of 121 MRSA patients compared with 123 MSSA patients, Graffunder et al. reported that MRSA-infected patients had a 1.5-fold longer postdiagnosis LOS than MSSA-infected patients (18). Ben-David et al. reported that in comparison to ICU patients with MSSA BSI, those with MRSA BSI had a higher median total hospital cost (US$42,137 vs. US$113,852), higher hospital cost after infection (US$17,603 vs. US$51,492), and greater LOS after infection (10.5 vs. 20.5 days). However, using a propensity score approach, the difference in cost after infection and the difference in LOS after infection for MRSA, compared with MSSA BSI, was not significant, suggesting the bivariate association was because of a confounding effect. Since the study was of limited size (76 ICU patients), definitive conclusions cannot be drawn but again indicate that future MRSA versus MSSA outcome analyses must account for potential confounders (59).

The methicillin resistance problem is not restricted to the acute care setting; it also significantly affects the costs associated with management of *S. aureus* surgical site infections (SA-SSI) (57), SA-BSI infections among community-dwelling hemodialysis-dependent patients (58), and MRSA infections in long-term care facilities (48). The median hospital cost was ~US$40,000 greater for patients with SSI because of MRSA (median, US$92,363; mean, US$118,415) than for patients with SSI because of MSSA (median, US$52,791; mean, US$73,165; $p < 0.001$). After adjusting for duration of surgery, length of hospitalization before infection, and comorbid conditions, methicillin resistance was found to be associated with a 1.19-fold increase in the median hospital cost ($p = 0.03$) and the mean cost per case attributable to methicillin resistance was US$13,901 per case of SA-SSI (58).

In a prospective study comparing MRSA among dialysis patients with MSSA bacteremic patients, adjusted costs were higher for patients with MRSA BSI for the initial hospitalization (US$21,251 vs. US$13,978, $p = 0.012$) and 12 weeks after the initial hospitalization (US$25,518 vs. US$17,354, p = 0.015) (58). Similarly, the median overall cost associated with MRSA infection in a long-term care facility was reported to be 1.95 times greater than that of MSSA infection (48). Although the magnitude of difference varies between investigations, studies have consistently demonstrated higher hospitalization costs and

LOS with MRSA when compared to MSSA infections, typically on the magnitude of 1.2- to 2.0-fold increase in morbidity and costs (47). The observed disparities in study results are most likely secondary to differences in study populations and costing structures. Collectively, these studies establish the gravity of MRSA compared to MSSA with respect to length of hospital stay and cost of hospitalization (10,18,22, 48,50,52,54,56–58).

CA-MRSA and Outcomes

It is important to recognize that the aforementioned MRSA outcomes studies did not distinguish between CA-MRSA and health care–associated HC-MRSA. Given the time frame of the studies, it is highly likely that the majority included patients with HC-MRSA. Because of the intrinsic differences in virulence, clinical presentation, antibiotic susceptibility, and at-risk populations between HC-MRSA and CA-MRSA, it is not possible to extrapolate the results from one MRSA strain to the other (27–45,61). The rising prevalence of CA-MRSA infections in both the community and hospital setting has prompted investigators to examine the outcomes specifically associated with both MRSA strains.

The majority of research examining the outcomes associated with CA-MRSA has focused on skin and soft-tissue infections (SSTIs) (29,45,46,62). The most comprehensive study to date is by Miller et al., which prospectively compared rehospitalization and 30-day post-discharge response rates among patients hospitalized with either a CA-MRSA or CA-MSSA SSTI (62). Interestingly, CA-MRSA-infected patients were *less* likely than CA-MSSA-infected patients to be rehospitalized during the 30 days after their initial hospitalization (4% vs. 23%, $p = 0.003$). Although rehospitalizations were more common among patients with CA-MSSA SSTIs, the 30-day postdischarge response rates were similar between patients with CA-MRSA and CA-MSSA SSTIs (33% vs. 28%, respectively, $p = 0.55$). Lack of incision and drainage was found to be the most important determinant of nonresponse at day 30 ($p = 0.005$), but other clinical factors, including receipt of inactive antibiotics, were not associated with failure.

The findings by Miller et al. do not coincide with other recent studies. In a prospective, multicenter evaluation of patients with community-associated *S. aureus* infections (over 85% of infections involved the skin/soft tissue), patients with CA-MRSA were less likely to achieve clinical cure when compared to CA-MSSA (61% vs. 84%, respectively, $p = 0.001$) (46). Patients with CA-MRSA infections had longer hospital stays (12 days vs. 10 days), recurrence or relapse (18% vs. 6%; $p < 0.015$), and higher rates of clinical failure (OR, 3.4; 95% CI, 1.7–6.9; $p < 0.001$). Although it was not the primary end point of this study, patients with CA-MRSA infections receiving active antimicrobial therapy were more likely to achieve clinical cure than those receiving inactive therapy. This finding is consistent with the study by Ruhe et al. (61), among CA-MRSA SSTIs. If an active antimicrobial agent was used within 48 hours of the first positive culture or first incision and drainage (time zero), there was a statistically significant positive impact on clinical outcome (95% vs. 87%).

Only one study to date has compared mortality rates between patients with CA-MRSA bacteremia and CA-MSSA bacteremia and this study was limited to patients with onset of *S. aureus* bacteremia within 48 hours of hospital presentation (63). Mortality was comparable between patients with CA-MRSA and CA-MSSA even though patients CA-MRSA infections were more likely to have necrotizing pneumonia and cutaneous abscesses.

Other Cost Considerations

It is important to note that the above morbidity and cost estimates are conservative and do not account for the additional costs incurred by implementing infection control measures. A Canadian study (64) undertook this analysis by including the cost for isolation and management of MRSA-colonized patients (estimated to be Can$1363 per admission) and the hospital's annual screening cost for MRSA was Can$109,813. Assuming a modest MRSA infection rate of 10% to 20%, they determined the cost associated with MRSA in Canadian hospitals to be Can$42 million to Can$59 million annually (64). This would be substantially higher if extrapolated to U.S. hospitals where the average MRSA rate is approximately 50% (7).

It is important to examine not only the cost of isolation and management of MRSA-colonized patients but the overall costs of MRSA screening. A study performed in a German hospital found that the screening expenditure for 539 patients over a 19-month period amounted to €26,241.51 (€16,573.58/yr) (65). These costs comprised €15,407.71 for medical consumables and €10,833.90 for additional nursing time. Clearly, screening costs should be considered in developing a total cost for MRSA diagnosis and treatment (66).

Most of these cost estimates do not account for the cost of managing MRSA infection outside the hospital, which may include the cost of rehabilitation, extended care facilities, or home IV therapy costs (67). Vancomycin can only be used intravenously to treat MRSA infection because the oral formulation is not absorbed. While it is beneficial to treat MRSA patients in the outpatient setting from the payer's standpoint, a recent study reported that the cost of drug acquisition, nursing time, supplies for outpatient IV vancomycin therapy, IV line placement, replacement and management costs, and laboratory costs were quite high and substantially more than the average daily reimbursement of approximately US$300 estimated from four different health care payers (67). None of these costs quantify the indirect costs or patient impact, which may include the emotional toll of having a drug-resistant infection, requiring a hospital isolation room, lost time from work for the patient and family because of a prolonged hospitalization and recovery period, and the long-term health consequences of having an MRSA infection (47).

FACTORS CONTRIBUTING TO MRSA IMPACT ON CLINICAL AND ECONOMIC OUTCOMES

The casual pathway for MRSA is complex, and the patient's outcome can be attributed to a confluence of factors related to the organism, treatment, and patient (47). While differences in fitness may explain differences in outcomes (68–72), several treatment-related factors provide a plausible explanation for the greater morbidity, mortality, and cost incurred by MRSA infections. At the time of organism identification and antibiotic susceptibility reporting, 32.9% of MRSA patients did not receive antibiotics that were microbiologically active against the MRSA BSI (73). An assessment of 398 patients with SA-BSI revealed that inappropriate empiric therapy was initiated in 141 patients (35.4%) with MRSA bacteremia (74), and in an outcomes study involving 353 patients, 42.9% of MRSA patients did not receive appropriate therapy within 45 hours of *S. aureus* bacteremia compared to only 9.8% of MSSA patients (51).

Numerous investigators in various practice settings have correlated the risk of a poor outcome to treatment delays (25,51,73–75). For patients with nosocomial SA-BSI, Lodise et al. (51) and others noted that patients with a treatment delay exceeding 45 hours were at an almost threefold higher risk of mortality compared to patients who received adequate antimicrobial therapy within 45 hours (25,26). The adjusted mean LOS was longer for patients with delayed treatment compared to those treated effectively within 45 hours of onset of BSI (20.2 days vs. 14.3 days, $p = 0.05$) (51). In an SA-BSI case-control study published recently, MRSA was significantly associated with infection-related mortality and 30-day mortality in the univariate analysis, but this relationship did not persist after adjustment for delayed appropriate treatment in the multivariate analyses. Delayed treatment was highly predictive of both infection-related mortality (OR, 2.2; 95% CI, 1.0–4.5; $p = 0.04$) and 30-day mortality (OR, 2.1; 95% CI, 1.0–4.5; $p = 0.04$) in the multivariate analyses (54). These studies underscore the importance of selecting the appropriate antibiotic early in the course of the infection and may partially explain the negative MRSA outcomes.

Beyond the complications caused by treatment delays, differences in antibiotics play a role in patient outcome for MRSA and MSSA. All of the studies above evaluated MRSA outcomes in the "vancomycin era." Although vancomycin remains the drug of choice for MRSA infections, it is not viewed as an optimal antibiotic by many clinicians on the basis of its data in serious MSSA infections (76). In vitro data indicate that vancomycin is actually inferior to the β-lactams with respect to the rate of bactericidal activity against MSSA (77), and clinical evidence suggests that the glycopeptides are inferior to β-lactam antibiotics as therapy for serious staphylococcal infections (17,49,78–81).

There are also emerging resistance concerns with vancomycin among MRSA infections Within the past 10 years, multiple reports have described MRSA strains with intermediate susceptibility or high-level resistance to vancomycin (72,82–86). Vancomycin resistance to *S. aureus* is underappreciated because the Clinical Laboratory Standard's Institute (CLSI) and Food and Drug Administration (FDA) susceptibility breakpoints are too high (MIC of ≤2 mg/L) (76). While most institutions have near 100% susceptibility to vancomycin, a shift to higher MIC values within the susceptibility range among MRSA isolates has been noted in several recent reports (87,88). This is concerning because data, albeit limited, suggest that vancomycin has reduced activity against MRSA infections with elevated vancomycin MIC values (87,89–92). Published data examining the relationship between vancomycin MIC values and MRSA infection outcomes have included a retrospective examination of dialysis patients with MRSA BSIs (91), a retrospective cohort study of patients with a mixed group of MRSA infections (90), and three observational cohort studies of patients with MRSA BSIs (87,92,93). Although the magnitude of differences were not as pronounced as the study by Sakoulas et al. (89), the results consistently demonstrated higher rates of failure, longer hospital stays, and increased mortality with MRSA infections with high MIC values when compared to MRSA infections with lower vancomycin MIC values. Collectively, these studies strongly suggest that serious MRSA infections with higher vancomycin MIC values do not respond as well to vancomycin as MRSA infections with lower vancomycin MIC values (87,89–93).

Comparative Studies Between Vancomycin and Recently Approved Agents with MRSA Activity

Limited data suggest newer MRSA agents may provide improved clinical and economic outcomes relative to vancomycin. The most robust data exist for linezolid (94,95). In a post hoc analysis of two prospective double-blind studies of patients with hospital-acquired pneumonia (96), clinical cure rates were significantly higher in the linezolid group compared to the vancomycin group (59.0% vs. 35.5%, $p < 0.01$), and this effect persisted in the logistic regression analysis (OR, 3.3; 95% CI, 1.3–8.3; $p = 0.01$) (95). The substandard clinical cure rates observed for vancomycin in these studies may be related to its inability to achieve sufficient concentration in the lungs and epithelial lining fluid (94,95).

A prospective pharmacoeconomic model was conducted to determine the incremental cost-effectiveness of linezolid compared with vancomycin for the treatment of VAP due to *S. aureus* (96). Investigators conducted a decision model analysis of the cost and efficacy of linezolid versus vancomycin. The primary outcome was the incremental cost-effectiveness of linezolid in terms of cost per added quality-adjusted life-year (QALY) gained. Model estimates were derived from prospective trials of linezolid for VAP and from other studies describing the costs and outcomes for VAP. Despite its higher cost, linezolid was cost-effective for treatment of VAP. The cost per QALY was approximately US$30,000. This is less than the accepted standard of US$100,000 per QALY for cost-effectiveness analysis in health care. The authors concluded that linezolid is a cost-effective alternative to vancomycin for the treatment of VAP.

In addition, linezolid has demonstrated higher clinical and micro-biologic success rates for MRSA surgical site infections and complicated SSTIs (cSSTI) (97,98). It is important to recognize that these linezolid versus vancomycin studies were not designed a priori to examine patients with MRSA infections, and interpretation of the results has been the subject of considerable debate (99). To address the design issues of the previous studies, a randomized, open-label, controlled, multicenter phase IV study was conducted comparing linezolid to vancomycin in the treatment of cSSTIs due to MRSA (100). This study included 537 patients randomized to linezolid and 515 to vancomycin, for a total of 1052. At the end of treatment, there was a statistically significant difference between linezolid and van-comycin (85.8% vs. 69.3%, respectively, $p < 0.001$). However, success at the end of study was comparable between the linezolid and vancomycin (83.2% vs. 79.5%, respectively, $p = 0.321$).

While clinical and microbiologic success appears to be more favor-able with linezolid relative to vancomycin for cSSTI, another demonstrated advantage is that linezolid is 100% bioavailable. The availability of anti-biotics with highly bioavailable oral formulations enables clinicians to switch their patients to oral dosing, thereby allowing the patient to be dis-charged earlier. A recent survey of internal medicine and infectious diseases doctors indicated that they would be more inclined to discharge MRSA patients earlier if a high-bioavailability oral formulation existed (101).

To determine the potential cost saving of an early switch to oral linezolid or early hospital discharge, Parodi et al. conducted a retrospective cohort study at the Veterans Administration Greater Los Angeles Healthcare System (102). Of the 172 patients who fulfilled the inclusion criteria, 103 (58.2%) were potentially eligible for switching to oral linezolid and 55 (32.0%) were eligible for early discharge. Investigators found that the mean savings per eligible treatment course in vancomycin therapy and LOS were 5.2 and 3.3 days, respectively, and the overall potential savings totaled US$220,181 with a mean savings per treatment course of US$4003. Examination of the economic outcomes of patients with known or suspected

MRSA infection treated with linezolid or vancomycin in phase III and IV trials has validated this position (97,98,103–107). McKinnon and colleagues observed a cost difference of US$1125 per patient in favor of linezolid (US$4881 vs. US$6006 for vancomycin-treated patients) when costs of drug, concomitant medications, procedures, and hospital costs were analyzed for the U.S. subset of patients with MRSA cSSTI (106).

Another antibiotic with promising activity against MRSA is daptomycin, which is a first-in-class lipopeptide antibiotic that is rapidly bactericidal against MRSA. It is approved for the treatment of cSSTI and SA-BSIs, including right-sided endocarditis, caused by MSSA and MRSA (108,109). Daptomycin performance was noninferior to the semisynthetic penicillins and vancomycin for cSSTI (108). A statistically significant 63% of the daptomycin-treated patients only required four to seven days of therapy, while 67% of those receiving a semisynthetic penicillin or vancomycin required therapy for at least eight days. A cSSTI prospective open-labeled study of daptomycin compared to historical control patients who received vancomycin revealed that patients treated with vancomycin also had significantly higher overall hospital costs (US$7,552) as compared to those treated with daptomycin (US$5,027) (110).

In the recent *S. aureus* bacteremia and endocarditis study comparing daptomycin to standard therapy (vancomycin or a β-lactam, both used in combination with a gentamicin for four days), comparable outcomes were observed, but with significantly less toxicity in the daptomycin group (109). A successful outcome was documented for 44.2% who received daptomycin compared to 41.7% who received standard therapy. Clinically significant renal dysfunction occurred in 11% of patients who received daptomycin and in 26% of patients who received standard therapy, emphasizing that even low-dose, short-duration gentamicin may have a dramatic effect on safety margins.

Bhavnani and colleagues performed an economic evaluation of the daptomycin bacteremia and endocarditis trial (111). They considered three cost strata: (*i*) the costs associated with drug acquisition; (*ii*) strata 1 costs plus costs for infusions, medications/procedures associated with drug-related adverse events, therapeutic drug monitoring, and treatment failures; and (*iii*) strata 1 and 2 costs plus hospital bed costs. When considering only the first two strata costs, the median cost-effectiveness ratios (C/E) were significantly higher for daptomcyin as compared to vancomycin. When hospital costs were included, the median C/E for daptomycin and vancomycin were statistically similar (US$23,639 vs. US$26,073). Interestingly, sensitivity analyses determined that if vancomycin was *free*, differences in aggregate median C/E ratios would not be statistically different.

Telavancin is another agent with activity against MRSA that has recently been approved by the FDA for cSSTIs. Telavancin is a semi-synthetic derivative of vancomycin with an added lipophilic component that is best characterized as a lipoglycopeptide (112). In two phase II cSSTI trials, a total of 93 patients infected with MRSA were studied. Of these, 89.6% in the telavancin group and 77.7% in the standard therapy group achieved cure (113,114). In phase III trials among patients with MRSA infections, cure rates were 91% among those receiving telavancin and 86% among patients receiving vancomycin (115). Laohavaleeson and colleagues performed an economic analysis of these phase III studies and determined that telavancin length of hospitalization and total costs were similar to those of vancomycin for the treatment of cSSTIs, particularly in those infected with MRSA (116). Although the findings for telavancin are promising, further study is needed to evaluate the impact of telavancin on patient outcomes and costs associated with MRSA infections. At the time of publication, there is no data confirming improved outcomes with tigecycline and quinupristin-dalfopristin for MRSA.

CONCLUSION

Rates of MRSA in the hospital and the community continue to increase. High patient morbidity, mortality, and resulting health care resource utilization are associated with MRSA when compared to MSSA. Studies evaluating the clinical and economic impact of MRSA compared to MSSA have consistently identified divergent patient outcomes. Although the data are not definitive, it appears that treatment-related factors may be primarily responsible for the negative outcomes observed with MRSA, as most studies demonstrating the negative patient outcomes and increased cost were performed when vancomycin was the mainstay of treatment for MRSA.

The role of vancomycin in the treatment of MRSA infections has recently been questioned, and there is a growing amount of clinical evidence that confirms the suboptimal response of MRSA to vancomycin, particularly for nosocomial pneumonia and SSTIs. Antibiotics with good bioavailability, such as linezolid, can facilitate early discharge and alleviate the economic burden of hospitalization for MRSA infections. In the era of newer agents such as linezolid, daptomycin, telavancin, and tigecycline, we will begin to learn more about the treatment-related factors, specifically antibiotic selection, that affect patient outcomes.

REFERENCES

1. Weinstein RA. Nosocomial infection update. Emerg Infect Dis 1998; 4(3): 416–420.
2. Jones RN. Resistance patterns among nosocomial pathogens: trends over the past few years. Chest 2001; 119(suppl 2):397S–404S.
3. Neu HC. The crisis in antibiotic resistance. Science 1992; 257(5073): 1064–1073.
4. Burton DC, Edwards JR, Horan TC, et al. Methicillin-resistant *Staphylococcus aureus* central line-associated bloodstream infections in US intensive care units, 1997–2007. JAMA 2009; 301(7):727–736.
5. Panlilio AL, Culver DH, Gaynes RP, et al. Methicillin-resistant *Staphylococcus aureus* in U.S. hospitals, 1975–1991. Infect Control Hosp Epidemiol 1992; 13(10):582–586.
6. Rosenthal VD, Maki DG, Mehta A, et al. International nosocomial infection control consortium report, data summary for 2002–2007, issued January 2008. Am J Infect Control 2008; 36(9):627–637.

7. National Nosocomial Infections Surveillance (NNIS) System Report, data summary from January 1992 through June 2004, issued October 2004. Am J Infect Control 2004; 32(8):470–485.

8. Hidron AI, Edwards JR, Patel J, et al. NHSN annual update: antimicrobial-resistant pathogens associated with healthcare-associated infections: annual summary of data reported to the national healthcare safety network at the centers for disease control and prevention, 2006–2007. Infect Control Hosp Epidemiol 2008; 29(11):996–1011.

9. Streit JM, Jones RN, Sader HS, et al. Assessment of pathogen occurrences and resistance profiles among infected patients in the intensive care unit: report from the SENTRY Antimicrobial Surveillance Program (North America, 2001). Int J Antimicrob Agents 2004; 24(2):111–118.

10. Abramson MA, Sexton DJ. Nosocomial methicillin-resistant and methicillin-susceptible *Staphylococcus aureus* primary bacteremia: at what costs? Infect Control Hosp Epidemiol 1999; 20(6):408–411.

11. Asensio A, Guerrero A, Quereda C, et al. Colonization and infection with methicillin-resistant *Staphylococcus aureus*: associated factors and eradication. Infect Control Hosp Epidemiol 1996; 17(1):20–28.

12. Blot SI, Vandewoude KH, Hoste EA, et al. Outcome and attributable mortality in critically Ill patients with bacteremia involving methicillin-susceptible and methicillin-resistant *Staphylococcus aureus*. Arch Intern Med 2002; 162(19):2229–2235.

13. Chang FY, MacDonald BB, Peacock JE Jr., et al. A prospective multicenter study of *Staphylococcus aureus* bacteremia: incidence of endocarditis, risk factors for mortality, and clinical impact of methicillin resistance. Medicine (Baltimore) 2003; 82(5):322–332.

14. Combes A, Luyt CE, Fagon JY, et al. Impact of methicillin resistance on outcome of *Staphylococcus aureus* ventilator-associated pneumonia. Am J Respir Crit Care Med 2004; 170(7):786–792.

15. Cosgrove SE, Sakoulas G, Perencevich EN, et al. Comparison of mortality associated with methicillin-resistant and methicillin-susceptible *Staphylococcus aureus* bacteremia: a meta-analysis. Clin Infect Dis 2003; 36(1):53–59.

16. Fowler VG, Jr., Olsen MK, Corey GR, et al. Clinical identifiers of complicated *Staphylococcus aureus* bacteremia. Arch Intern Med 2003; 163(17): 2066–2072.

17. Gonzalez C, Rubio M, Romero-Vivas J, et al. Bacteremic pneumonia due to *Staphylococcus aureus*: a comparison of disease caused by methicillin-resistant and methicillin-susceptible organisms. Clin Infect Dis 1999; 29(5):1171–1177.

18. Graffunder EM, Venezia RA. Risk factors associated with nosocomial methicillin-resistant *Staphylococcus aureus* (MRSA) infection including previous use of antimicrobials. J Antimicrob Chemother 2002; 49(6): 999–1005.

19. Hershow RC, Khayr WF, Smith NL. A comparison of clinical virulence of nosocomially acquired methicillin-resistant and methicillin-sensitive *Staphylococcus aureus* infections in a university hospital. Infect Control Hosp Epidemiol 1992; 13(10):587–593.

20. Harbarth S, Rutschmann O, Sudre P, et al. Impact of methicillin resistance on the outcome of patients with bacteremia caused by *Staphylococcus aureus*. Arch Intern Med 1998; 158(2):182–189.

21. Lodise TP Jr., McKinnon PS, Rybak M. Prediction model to identify patients with *Staphylococcus aureus* bacteremia at risk for methicillin resistance. Infect Control Hosp Epidemiol 2003; 24(9):655–661.

22. McHugh CG, Riley LW. Risk factors and costs associated with methicillin-resistant *Staphylococcus aureus* bloodstream infections. Infect Control Hosp Epidemiol 2004; 25(5):425–30.

23. Melzer M, Eykyn SJ, Gransden WR, et al. Is methicillin-resistant *Staphylococcus aureus* more virulent than methicillin-susceptible *S. aureus*? A comparative cohort study of British patients with nosocomial infection and bacteremia. Clin Infect Dis 2003; 37(11):1453–1460.

24. Peacock JE Jr., Moorman DR, Wenzel RP, et al. Methicillin-resistant *Staphylococcus aureus*: microbiologic characteristics, antimicrobial susceptibilities, and assessment of virulence of an epidemic strain. J Infect Dis 1981; 144(6):575–582.

25. Romero-Vivas J, Rubio M, Fernandez C, et al. Mortality associated with nosocomial bacteremia due to methicillin-resistant *Staphylococcus aureus*. Clin Infect Dis 1995; 21(6):1417–1423.

26. Soriano A, Martinez JA, Mensa J, et al. Pathogenic significance of methicillin resistance for patients with *Staphylococcus aureus* bacteremia. Clin Infect Dis 2000; 30(2):368–373.

27. Ochoa TJ, Mohr J, Wanger A, et al. Community-associated methicillin-resistant *Staphylococcus aureus* in pediatric patients. Emerg Infect Dis 2005; 11(6):966–968.

28. Harbarth S, Francois P, Shrenzel J, et al. Community-associated methicillin-resistant *Staphylococcus aureus*, Switzerland. Emerg Infect Dis 2005; 11(6): 962–965.

29. Moran GJ, Amii RN, Abrahamian FM, et al. Methicillin-resistant *Staphylococcus aureus* in community-acquired skin infections. Emerg Infect Dis 2005; 11(6):928–930.

30. Mulvey MR, MacDougall L, Cholin B, et al. Community-associated methicillin-resistant *Staphylococcus aureus*, Canada. Emerg Infect Dis 2005; 11(6):844–850.

31. Lee NE, Taylor MM, Bancroft E, et al. Risk factors for community-associated methicillin-resistant *Staphylococcus aureus* skin infections among HIV-positive men who have sex with men. Clin Infect Dis 2005; 40(10):1529–1534.

32. Nguyen DM, Mascola L, Brancoft E. Recurring methicillin-resistant *Staphylococcus aureus* infections in a football team. Emerg Infect Dis 2005; 11(4):526–532.

33. Ribeiro A, Dias C, Silva-Carvalho MC, et al. First report of infection with community-acquired methicillin-resistant *Staphylococcus aureus* in South America. J Clin Microbiol 2005; 43(4):1985–1988.

34. Kazakova SV, Hageman JC, Matava M, et al. A clone of methicillin-resistant *Staphylococcus aureus* among professional football players. N Engl J Med 2005; 352(5):468–875.

35. Baillargeon J, Kelley MF, Leach CT, et al. Methicillin-resistant *Staphylococcus aureus* infection in the Texas prison system. Clin Infect Dis 2004; 38(9): e92–e95.

36. Pan ES, Diep BA, Carleton HA, et al. Increasing prevalence of methicillin-resistant *Staphylococcus aureus* infection in California jails. Clin Infect Dis 2003; 37(10):1384–1388.

37. Methicillin-resistant *Staphylococcus aureus* infections in correctional facilities—Georgia, California, and Texas, 2001–2003. MMWR Morb Mortal Wkly Rep 2003; 52(41):992–996.

38. Methicillin-resistant *Staphylococcus aureus* skin or soft tissue infections in a state prison—Mississippi, 2000. MMWR Morb Mortal Wkly Rep 2001; 50(42):919–922.

39. Shukla SK, Stemper ME, Ramaswamy SV, et al. Molecular characteristics of nosocomial and Native American community-associated methicillin-resistant *Staphylococcus aureus* clones from rural Wisconsin. J Clin Microbiol 2004; 42(8):3752–3757.

40. Naimi TS, LeDell KH, Como-Sabetti K, et al. Comparison of community- and health care-associated methicillin-resistant *Staphylococcus aureus* infection. JAMA 2003; 290(22):2976–2984.

41. Rybak MJ, Pharm DK. Community-associated methicillin-resistant *Staphylococcus aureus*: a review. Pharmacotherapy 2005; 25(1):74–85.
42. Fridkin SK, Hageman JC, Morrison M, et al. Methicillin-resistant *Staphylococcus aureus* disease in three communities. N Engl J Med 2005; 352(14): 1436–1444.
43. Como-Sabetti K, Harriman KH, Buck JM, et al. Community-associated methicillin-resistant *Staphylococcus aureus*: trends in case and isolate characteristics from six years of prospective surveillance. Public Health Rep 2009; 124(3):427–435.
44. Maree CL, Daum RS, Boyle-Vavra S, et al. Community-associated methicillin-resistant *Staphylococcus aureus* isolates causing healthcare-associated infections. Emerg Infect Dis 2007; 13(2):236–242.
45. Klevens RM, Morrison MA, Nadle J, et al. Invasive methicillin-resistant *Staphylococcus aureus* infections in the United States. JAMA 2007; 298(15): 1763–1771.
46. Davis SL, Perri MB, Donabedian SM, et al. Epidemiology and outcomes of community-associated methicillin-resistant *Staphylococcus aureus* infection. J Clin Microbiol 2007; 45(6):1705–1711.
47. Cosgrove SE, Carmeli Y. The impact of antimicrobial resistance on health and economic outcomes. Clin Infect Dis 2003; 36(11):1433–1437.
48. Capitano B, Leshem OA, Nightingale CH, et al. Cost effect of managing methicillin-resistant *Staphylococcus aureus* in a long-term care facility. J Am Geriatr Soc 2003; 51(1):10–16.
49. Chang FY, Peacock JE Jr., Musher DM, et al. *Staphylococcus aureus* bacteremia: recurrence and the impact of antibiotic treatment in a prospective multicenter study. Medicine (Baltimore) 2003; 82(5):333–339.
50. Cosgrove SE, Qi Y, Kaye KS, et al. The impact of methicillin resistance in *Staphylococcus aureus* bacteremia on patient outcomes: mortality, length of stay, and hospital charges. Infect Control Hosp Epidemiol 2005; 26(2):166–174.
51. Lodise TP, McKinnon PS, Swiderski L, et al. Outcomes analysis of delayed antibiotic treatment for hospital-acquired *Staphylococcus aureus* bacteremia. Clin Infect Dis 2003; 36(11):1418–1423.
52. Rubin RJ, Harrington CA, Poon A, et al. The economic impact of *Staphylococcus aureus* infection in New York City hospitals. Emerg Infect Dis 1999; 5(1):9–17.
53. Whitby M, McLaws ML, Berry G. Risk of death from methicillin-resistant *Staphylococcus aureus* bacteraemia: a meta-analysis. Med J Aust 2001; 175(5):264–267.

54. Lodise TP, McKinnon PS. Clinical and economic impact of methicillin resistance in patients with *Staphylococcus aureus* bacteremia. Diagn Microbiol Infect Dis 2005; 52(2):113–122.

55. Athanassa Z, Siempos II, Falagas ME. Impact of methicillin resistance on mortality in *Staphylococcus aureus* VAP: a systematic review. Eur Respir J 2008; 31(3):625–632.

56. Wakefield DS, Helms CM, Massanari RM, et al. Cost of nosocomial infection: relative contributions of laboratory, antibiotic, and per diem costs in serious *Staphylococcus aureus* infections. Am J Infect Control 1988; 16(5):185–192.

57. Engemann JJ, Carmeli Y, Cosgrove SE, et al. Adverse clinical and economic outcomes attributable to methicillin resistance among patients with *Staphylococcus aureus* surgical site infection. Clin Infect Dis 2003; 36(5): 592–498.

58. Reed SD, Friedman JY, Engemann JJ, et al. Costs and outcomes among hemodialysis-dependent patients with methicillin-resistant or methicillin-susceptible *Staphylococcus aureus* bacteremia. Infect Control Hosp Epidemiol 2005; 26(2):175–183.

59. Ben-David D, Novikov I, Mermel LA. Are there differences in hospital cost between patients with nosocomial methicillin-resistant *Staphylococcus aureus* bloodstream infection and those with methicillin-susceptible *S. aureus* bloodstream infection? Infect Control Hosp Epidemiol 2009; 30(5):453–460.

60. Shorr AF, Tabak YP, Gupta V, et al. Morbidity and cost burden of methicillin-resistant *Staphylococcus aureus* in early onset ventilator-associated pneumonia. Crit Care 2006; 10(3):R97.

61. Ruhe JJ, Smith N, Bradsher RW, et al. Community-onset methicillin-resistant *Staphylococcus aureus* skin and soft-tissue infections: impact of antimicrobial therapy on outcome. Clin Infect Dis 2007; 44(6):777–784.

62. Miller LG, Quan C, Shay A, et al. A prospective investigation of outcomes after hospital discharge for endemic, community-acquired methicillin-resistant and -susceptible *Staphylococcus aureus* skin infection. Clin Infect Dis 2007; 44(4):483–492.

63. Wang JL, Chen SY, Wang JT, et al. Comparison of both clinical features and mortality risk associated with bacteremia due to community-acquired methicillin-resistant *Staphylococcus aureus* and methicillin-susceptible *S. aureus*. Clin Infect Dis 2008; 46(6):799–806.

64. Kim T, Oh PI, Simor AE. The economic impact of methicillin-resistant *Staphylococcus aureus* in Canadian hospitals. Infect Control Hosp Epidemiol 2001; 22(2):99–104.

65. Wernitz MH, Keck S, Swidsinski S, et al. Cost analysis of a hospital-wide selective screening programme for methicillin-resistant *Staphylococcus aureus* (MRSA) carriers in the context of diagnosis related groups (DRG) payment. Clin Microbiol Infect 2005; 11(6):466–471.

66. McGinigle KL, Gourlay ML, Buchanan IB. The use of active surveillance cultures in adult intensive care units to reduce methicillin-resistant *Staphylococcus aureus*-related morbidity, mortality, and costs: a systematic review. Clin Infect Dis 2008; 46(11):1717–1725.

67. Tice AD, Hoaglund PA, Nolet B, et al. Cost perspectives for outpatient intravenous antimicrobial therapy. Pharmacotherapy 2002; 22(2 pt 2):63S–70S.

68. Fowler VG Jr., Sakoulas G, McIntyre LM, et al. Persistent bacteremia due to methicillin-resistant *Staphylococcus aureus* infection is associated with agr dysfunction and low-level in vitro resistance to thrombin-induced platelet microbicidal protein. J Infect Dis 2004; 190(6):1140–1149.

69. Moise-Broder PA, Sakoulas G, Eliopoulos GM, et al. Accessory gene regulator group II polymorphism in methicillin-resistant *Staphylococcus aureus* is predictive of failure of vancomycin therapy. Clin Infect Dis 2004; 38(12): 1700–1705.

70. Sakoulas G, Eliopoulos GM, Moellering RC Jr., et al. *Staphylococcus aureus* accessory gene regulator (agr) group II: is there a relationship to the development of intermediate-level glycopeptide resistance? J Infect Dis 2003; 187(6):929–938.

71. Sakoulas G, Eliopoulos GM, Moellering RC Jr., et al. Accessory gene regulator (agr) locus in geographically diverse *Staphylococcus aureus* isolates with reduced susceptibility to vancomycin. Antimicrob Agents Chemother 2002; 46(5):1492–1502.

72. Sakoulas G, Moellering RC Jr., Eliopoulos GM. Adaptation of methicillin-resistant *Staphylococcus aureus* in the face of vancomycin therapy. Clin Infect Dis 2006; 42(suppl 1):S40–S50.

73. Ibrahim EH, Sherman G, Ward S, et al. The influence of inadequate antimicrobial treatment of bloodstream infections on patient outcomes in the ICU setting. Chest 2000; 118(1):146–155.

74. Leibovici L, Shraga I, Drucker M, et al. The benefit of appropriate empirical antibiotic treatment in patients with bloodstream infection. J Intern Med 1998; 244(5):379–386.

75. Kollef MH, Ward S, Sherman G, et al. Inadequate treatment of nosocomial infections is associated with certain empiric antibiotic choices. Crit Care Med 2000; 28(10):3456–3464.

76. Tenover FC, Moellering RC Jr. The rationale for revising the Clinical and Laboratory Standards Institute vancomycin minimal inhibitory concentration interpretive criteria for *Staphylococcus aureus*. Clin Infect Dis 2007; 44(9):1208–1215.

77. Cantoni L, Glauser MP, Bille J. Comparative efficacy of daptomycin, vancomycin, and cloxacillin for the treatment of *Staphylococcus aureus* endocarditis in rats and role of test conditions in this determination. Antimicrob Agents Chemother 1990; 34(12):2348–2353.

78. Levine DP, Fromm BS, Reddy BR. Slow response to vancomycin or vancomycin plus rifampin in methicillin-resistant *Staphylococcus aureus* endocarditis. Ann Intern Med 1991; 115(9):674–680.

79. Small PM, Chambers HF. Vancomycin for *Staphylococcus aureus* endocarditis in intravenous drug users. Antimicrob Agents Chemother 1990; 34(6):1227–1231.

80. Lodise TP Jr., McKinnon PS, Levine DP, et al. Impact of empirical-therapy selection on outcomes of intravenous drug users with infective endocarditis caused by methicillin-susceptible *Staphylococcus aureus*. Antimicrob Agents Chemother 2007; 51(10):3731–3733.

81. Fowler VG Jr., Kong LK, Corey GR, et al. Recurrent *Staphylococcus aureus* bacteremia: pulsed-field gel electrophoresis findings in 29 patients. J Infect Dis 1999; 179(5):1157–1161.

82. Whitener CJ, Park SY, Browne FA, et al. Vancomycin-resistant *Staphylococcus aureus* in the absence of vancomycin exposure. Clin Infect Dis 2004; 38(8):1049–1055.

83. Centers for Disease Control and Prevention (CDC). *Staphylococcus aureus* resistant to vancomycin—United States, 2002. MMWR Morb Mortal Wkly Rep 2002; 51(26):565–567.

84. Centers for Disease Control and Prevention (CDC). Vancomycin-resistant *Staphylococcus aureus*—Pennsylvania, 2002. MMWR Morb Mortal Wkly Rep 2002; 51(40):902.

85. Sievert DM, Rudrik JT, Patel JB, et al. Vancomycin-resistant *Staphylococcus aureus* in the United States, 2002–2006. Clin Infect Dis 2008; 46(5): 668–674.

86. Finks J, Wells E, Dyke TL, et al. Vancomycin-resistant *Staphylococcus aureus*, Michigan, USA, 2007. Emerg Infect Dis 2009; 15(6):943–945.

87. Lodise TP, Graves J, Evans A, et al. Relationship between vancomycin MIC and failure among patients with methicillin-resistant *Staphylococcus aureus* bacteremia treated with vancomycin. Antimicrob Agents Chemother 2008; 52(9):3315–3320.

88. Steinkraus G, White R, Friedrich L. Vancomycin MIC creep in non-vancomycin-intermediate *Staphylococcus aureus* (VISA), vancomycin-susceptible clinical methicillin-resistant *S. aureus* (MRSA) blood isolates from 2001 05. J Antimicrob Chemother 2007; 60(4):788–794.

89. Sakoulas G, Moise-Broder PA, Schentag J, et al. Relationship of MIC and bactericidal activity to efficacy of vancomycin for treatment of methicillin-resistant *Staphylococcus aureus* bacteremia. J Clin Microbiol 2004; 42(6): 2398–2402.

90. Hidayat LK, Hsu DI, Quist R, et al. High-dose vancomycin therapy for methicillin-resistant *Staphylococcus aureus* infections: efficacy and toxicity. Arch Intern Med 2006; 166(19):2138–2144.

91. Maclayton DO, Suda KJ, Coval KA, et al. Case-control study of the relationship between MRSA bacteremia with a vancomycin MIC of 2 microg/mL and risk factors, costs, and outcomes in inpatients undergoing hemodialysis. Clin Ther 2006; 28(8):1208–1216.

92. Soriano A, Marco F, Martinez JA, et al. Influence of vancomycin minimum inhibitory concentration on the treatment of methicillin-resistant *Staphylococcus aureus* bacteremia. Clin Infect Dis 2008; 46(2):193–200.

93. Musta AC, Riederer K, Shemes S, et al. Vancomycin MIC plus heteroresistance and outcome of methicillin-resistant *Staphylococcus aureus* bacteremia: trends over 11 years. J Clin Microbiol 2009; 47(6): 1640–1644.

94. Cruciani M, Gatti G, Lazzarini L, et al. Penetration of vancomycin into human lung tissue. J Antimicrob Chemother 1996; 38(5):865–869.

95. Lamer C, de Beco V, Soler P, et al. Analysis of vancomycin entry into pulmonary lining fluid by bronchoalveolar lavage in critically ill patients. Antimicrob Agents Chemother 1993; 37(2):281–286.

96. Shorr AF, Susla GM, Kollef MH. Linezolid for treatment of ventilator-associated pneumonia: a cost-effective alternative to vancomycin. Crit Care Med 2004; 32(1):137–143.

97. Weigelt J, Itani K, Stevens D, et al. Linezolid versus vancomycin in treatment of complicated skin and soft tissue infections. Antimicrob Agents Chemother 2005; 49(6):2260–2266.

98. Weigelt J, Kaafarani HM, Itani KM, et al. Linezolid eradicates MRSA better than vancomycin from surgical-site infections. Am J Surg 2004; 188(6): 760–766.

99. Powers JH, Ross DB, Lin D, et al. Linezolid and vancomycin for methicillin-resistant *Staphylococcus aureus* nosocomial pneumonia: the subtleties of subgroup analyses. Chest 2004; 126(1):314–315; author reply 5–6.

100. Itani K, Weigelt J, Stevens D, et al. Efficacy and safety of linezolid versus vancomycin for the treatment of complicated skin and soft-tissue infections proven to be due to meticillin resistant *Staphylococcus aureus*. Abstract #O80. 18th European Congress of Clinical Microbiology and Infectious Diseases Barcelona, Spain, April 19–22, 2008.

101. Yaldo AZ, Sullivan JL, Li Z. Factors influencing physicians' decision to discharge hospitalized patients infected with methicillin-resistant *Staphylococcus aureus*. Am J Health-Syst Pharm 2001; 58(18):1756–1759.

102. Parodi S, Rhew DC, Goetz MB. Early switch and early discharge opportunities in intravenous vancomycin treatment of suspected methicillin-resistant staphylococcal species infections. J Manag Care Pharm 2003; 9(4): 317–326.

103. Li JZ, Willke RJ, Rittenhouse BE, et al. Approaches to analysis of length of hospital stay related to antibiotic therapy in a randomized clinical trial: linezolid versus vancomycin for treatment of known or suspected methicillin-resistant *Staphylococcus* species infections. Pharmacotherapy 2002; 22(2 Pt 2):45S–54S.

104. Li JZ, Willke RJ, Rittenhouse BE, et al. Effect of linezolid versus vancomycin on length of hospital stay in patients with complicated skin and soft tissue infections caused by known or suspected methicillin-resistant staphylococci: results from a randomized clinical trial. Surg Infect (Larchmt) 2003; 4(1):57–70.

105. Li Z, Willke RJ, Pinto LA, et al. Comparison of length of hospital stay for patients with known or suspected methicillin-resistant *Staphylococcus* species infections treated with linezolid or vancomycin: a randomized, multicenter trial. Pharmacotherapy 2001; 21(3):263–274.

106. McKinnon PS, Sorensen SV, Liu LZ, et al. Impact of linezolid on economic outcomes and determinants of cost in a clinical trial evaluating patients with MRSA complicated skin and soft-tissue infections. Ann Pharmacother 2006; 40(6):1017–1023.

107. Itani KM, Weigelt J, Li JZ, et al. Linezolid reduces length of stay and duration of intravenous treatment compared with vancomycin for

complicated skin and soft tissue infections due to suspected or proven methicillin-resistant *Staphylococcus aureus* (MRSA). Int J Antimicrob Agents 2005; 26(6):442–448.

108. Arbeit RD, Maki D, Tally FP, et al. The safety and efficacy of daptomycin for the treatment of complicated skin and skin-structure infections. Clin Infect Dis 2004; 38(12):1673–1681.

109. Fowler VG Jr., Boucher HW, Corey GR, et al. Daptomycin versus standard therapy for bacteremia and endocarditis caused by *Staphylococcus aureus*. N Engl J Med 2006; 355(7):653–665.

110. Davis SL, McKinnon PS, Hall LM, et al. Daptomycin versus vancomycin for complicated skin and skin structure infections: clinical and economic outcomes. Pharmacotherapy 2007; 27(12):1611–1618.

111. Bhavnani SM, Prakhya A, Hammel JP, et al. Cost-effectiveness of daptomycin and vancomycin in patients with methicillin-resistant *Staphylococcus aureus* bacteremia and/or endocarditis. Clin Infect Dis 2009; 49(5):691–698.

112. Leonard SN, Rybak MJ. Telavancin: an antimicrobial with a multifunctional mechanism of action for the treatment of serious gram-positive infections. Pharmacotherapy 2008; 28(4):458–468.

113. Stryjewski ME, Chu VH, O'Riordan WD, et al. Telavancin versus standard therapy for treatment of complicated skin and skin structure infections caused by gram-positive bacteria: FAST 2 study. Antimicrob Agents Chemother 2006; 50(3):862–867.

114. Stryjewski ME, O'Riordan WD, Lau WK, et al. Telavancin versus standard therapy for treatment of complicated skin and soft-tissue infections due to gram-positive bacteria. Clin Infect Dis 2005; 40(11):1601–1607.

115. Wilson SE, O'Riordan W, Hopkins A, et al. Telavancin versus vancomycin for the treatment of complicated skin and skin-structure infections associated with surgical procedures. Am J Surg 2009; 197(6):791–796.

116. Laohavaleeson S, Barriere SL, Nicolau DP, et al. Cost-effectiveness of telavancin versus vancomycin for treatment of complicated skin and skin structure infections. Pharmacotherapy 2008; 28(12):1471–1482.

Index

Milton Keynes UK
Ingram Content Group UK Ltd.
UKHW022048141024
449569UK00031B/1545